AN OSTEOPATHIC ODYSSEY

Third Edition

James Jealous D.O.

Edited by Jennifer Weiss, D.O.

Disclaimer

The material in this book is for informational purposes only; it is not intended as a substitute for the advice and care of your health practitioner. The author and copyright holder especially disclaimed responsibility for any decisions, actions, or effects that may result from reliance upon the use and application of the material.

This book is dedicated to the eternal memory of
Dr Still.
He began a Tidal Wave of Service.

For more information about Dr. Jealous please visit:
https://BiodynamicsOfOsteopathy.com

AN OSTEOPATHIC ODYSSEY

Hardback ISBN: 979-8-2957-5044-1

First Edition November 2015
Second Edition April 2024
Third Edition March 2026

The World Is Too Much With Us

The world is too much with us; late and soon,
Getting and spending, we lay waste our powers;—
Little we see in Nature that is ours;
We have given our hearts away, a sordid boon!
This Sea that bares her bosom to the moon;
The winds that will be howling at all hours,
And are up-gathered now like sleeping flowers;
For this, for everything, we are out of tune;
It moves us not. Great God! I'd rather be
A Pagan suckled in a creed outworn;
So might I, standing on this pleasant lea,
Have glimpses that would make me less forlorn;
Have sight of Proteus rising from the sea;
Or hear old Triton blow his wreathèd horn.

William Wordsworth

PREFACE

This is not a textbook. It is the travelogue of one man who has tried to become an Osteopath. Osteopathy has been a part of my life since my birth in 1943 at the Osteopathic Hospital in Saco, Maine. My dad was a D.O. as was my godfather. Through them, while still a young man, I met many well-known Osteopaths.

When my father died in 1957, I was 14. I began working as an x-ray technician in the local Osteopathic hospital. I enjoyed the cohesiveness of a profession trying to survive its growth. I lived for many years inside a flourishing profession.

I entered Kirksville in 1965. The class was riddled with students who just wanted to be doctors and had little respect for Osteopathic principles, but the faculty and hospital staff were absolutely alive with skilled hands and listening hearts. Traditional Osteopathy was practiced. Any interested student could easily find many mentors who were exceptional.

While I had many influential and skilled professors, I want to speak of my experience with George Laughlin, the grandson of A.T. Still. I first entered his office as a second year student. I was attired in my white coat carrying a black bag that had some essential tools inside. Dr. Laughlin was a strong personality with a big heart. For those who wanted real Osteopathy he was a beacon. The first patient that day had obstructive lung disease and was oxygen dependent. Dr. Laughlin greeted him like an old friend, as he did all his patients. I liked his lack of self-importance and his obvious love for humanity.

I sat in the corner of the treatment room, my bag beside me, and watched. The patient removed the oxygen tube from his nose — I was already worrying he would collapse. Then Dr. Laughlin had him lie down with his head slightly elevated.

I expected to see myofascial release and rib-raising, among other techniques, applied to reduce the restrictions and increase flow. I was on the edge of my seat ready to see a master at work.

Dr. Laughlin delicately placed his hands under the patient's head and neck. The doctor's head bowed slightly as he became extremely still ... his eyes closed. I was dumbfounded. What was he doing?

He was not moving tissue. I thought maybe he was tired and had fallen asleep but...the patient's face was showing pink skin, a gross change from the grayish coloration he had had when he entered the room. I could not believe what I was seeing! How was this possible? Dr. Laughlin remained statuesque. I was blank.

The patient's diaphragm was easing and the travail of breathing and suffering were fading before my eyes. Dr. George was still seemingly immobile.

His skill disarmed me of all of the knowledge I thought my education had given me. The patient got up and left ... not using his oxygen. Dr. Laughlin said that the patient would have several days of freedom from the oxygen but that the main goal was to keep what potential health he had at a maximum.

Though it made sense to me, I also realized how insane his approach would appear to many Allopaths and Osteopaths alike. Still said, in many more words, *you judge an Osteopath by his results, not what he says*[1]. Dr. Laughlin sat for a moment with me; I felt blessed and aware that Osteopathy was not what the AOA dictates. I felt calm. I felt safe with him as a person and a mentor. I liked his 'country doctor' style and his generous use of time. The Osteopathic oath says, " I will be a friend to my patients." I admired this aspect of the Osteopathic physicians I met and saw it clearly in Dr. Laughlin. It was so unlike the sterile 'holier-than-thou' attitude and coldness many physicians projected. I knew then that I would be a country doctor. Now, forty-eight years later, I know I felt the higher presence of Osteopathy in that room.

---

1 Still Page 19 Philosophy and Principles of Osteopathy. See also Bibliography and Notes

I remember little of Dr. Laughlin's words from that time. I was with him in a way that felt like an initiation into a legacy. Now I know that the greatest teachers spoke as much in silence as they did in words. What you received depended on what you heard of both.
But there is more that you, the reader, have directly received from Dr. Laughlin.

In 1953 The AOA outlawed Sutherland's work and blackmailed all Osteopathic Colleges. Since all Osteopathic medical schools were dependent on the AOA for accreditation, teaching Sutherland's work meant risking accreditation privileges. All the colleges were afraid of the ruling and complied—except Kirksville. George Laughlin wrote the AOA and stated that he was personally having a course at the school, and if they wanted they could come and close Kirksville. He recruited help, though it was hard to find, as most Osteopaths who came feared they might lose their license, as well as face personal consequences. The only people to help him were Anne Wales, Chester Handy, Ruby Day and Dr. Quint. Three of them came from New England, and it took two weeks by boat from Boston via the Mississippi River. George paid the cost for the faculty and for the eleven students who came. The course went on and the AOA was silent. Without his effort cranial work would have ended right then.

Think about what we owe these souls! We are blessed to have found the legacy of those who remained in spite of great adversarial forces.

Over many years I have also seen the gross destruction of our hospitals and schools by Allopathic institutions that have left the profession with few natural resources. Osteopathy today is dying. Even though the bones remain, the art of our tradition is fading with the cloaking of Osteopathy in academic reductionism. Many see this paralysis in our organizations, and yet around the edges there flourishes a community of love and wholeness that "digs on"[1] into the luminous night of the not yet known.[2]

1 Sutherland see Bibliography and Notes
2 see Bibliography and Notes

Osteopathy is kept intact by artistry, scientific thinking, and a loving legacy. This legacy has been passed, uninterrupted from Dr. Still to my teachers. For myself, this treasure was given to me by George Laughlin, Ruby Day, Rollin Becker, Alan Becker, Anne Wales, and many unnoted people.

I have learned from them. I have also spent a lifetime in the wilderness learning how to heal myself and help others through observation of natural laws.

This is the authority under which I write and speak. It is not mine but an extension of the lifetime of many doctors who have taken up the general practice of Osteopathy as prescribed by our oral tradition. It is a deep moving love that builds daily and proves that the magnitude of Osteopathy will live on.

As we sit together in joy, let us be thankful for the greatness of Osteopathy that has survived, for the open secret of the Master Mechanic who is close at hand and breathing. for the love that binds our wounds and our community.[1]

This book is designed by the Tide. The divisions and order are spontaneous and may seem irrational. I hope it is an enjoyable task to use this book as a 'friend' to be with you.

Jennifer Weiss, D.O. Has worked very hard to make sure all this came together in a timely and clear fashion. If you like what we have done please thank her.

James Jealous, DO
April 25th 2015
Talent Oregon

1 See Bibliography and Notes

An Osteopathic Odyssey

THE ART OF OSTEOPATHY January 1

"We must learn to communicate and cooperate with natural laws, not framed by human hands."[1]

These words have been handed down to us from Dr. Still, Dr. Sutherland and their closest students. This is the art of Osteopathy: to perceive natural laws expressing involuntary motion, inherent order, and intention. The mind must remain detached for long periods of time. In this state the mind can watch natural laws at work. One can, with repeated study, see relationships and landscapes. The art of Osteopathy is what we learn in these observations.

The science of Osteopathy emerges from the art as one observes the order and meaning of natural laws expressed over and over in a variety of patients. The repetition of landscapes reveals the laws.

To sit in the woods with no purpose other than sitting brings on stage a world unseen by the routine of the cultural persona. Dr. Still lived in this simplicity. His writings reflect his search for answers and the call to service.

1 Sutherland page 300 COT quoting Still Page 302 Autobiography

THERAPEUTIC FORCES

January 2

"All one does is begin a treatment." [1]

"I bind the wound, God heals it." [2]

Many of my teachers in Kirksville made the statement, "all you do is begin a treatment, then the indwelling therapeutic forces finish it."

The goal, of engaging an indwelling therapeutic, process is the hallmark of our tradition.

This is not an ideology but a directly perceived reality that one begins to appreciate by following the therapeutic forces and accepting the wisdom behind the amount and direction of treatment. One must give up prioritizing by formulation and learn the deeper science of knowing the movements of life.

Knowing the mechanism of life is not a willy-nilly going with the flow ... not at all; it is the result of long and disciplined experience.

The idea of doing a treatment to the patient with your intelligence and intention eventually dies ... in my case it was twenty years and 80,000 treatments ... and then another ten years of becoming neutral to the intuition which tried to preempt the Tide.

Then it began.

Over time we grow in our skill and patience. Early on we find there is an ego need to be certain that one is intelligent, intuitive and free. Then we come to an interior room where we are a guest and a beginner ... here we learn to trust the Tide and as we do, we begin to see Osteopathy in a very different light.When you feel this journey takes too long think about the service that we are doing. You will slowly see that eternity is not a long time—it is no time at all. You are not alone you are a branch on the tree of Osteopathy nourished by all that has been since the seed fell and opened to the sun.

---

1 Becker see Bibliography and Notes

2 Galen, Greek physician AD 129 – c. 200/c. 216, see also Bibliography and Notes

BECOMING A BEGINNER January 3

The Tide never does the same thing, the same way, twice; neither does a master.

It is tempting to try and repeat the steps from a successful treatment.

We see results, then reflect back on the nature of the treatment and try to reproduce the process. The process, if one looks closely, was dispensed by the Tide. The Tide never repeats a procedure exactly in the same manner—never. We must be honest enough to see who gave the treatment and correct our center stage rewrites where we play a central role.

Commit to a new beginning with each patient. Then the Teacher will demonstrate a fresh teaching.

Essentially there are no techniques, only Principles. You will have great joy from seeing the ever-changing vistas under your hands and the service to humanity that the Tide orchestrates everywhere.

MOTHER NATURE January 4

"This is not an idle dream."[1]

This statement by Dr. Sutherland needs repeating more today than in his era. The wisdom of Mother Nature is smothered by the rapid pace of our lives. Sunrise and sunset do not mean anything anymore. We do not feel them. We are so full that we have no room for the small quiet motions of life and the essential slow flow of the feminine.

Mother Nature is not a fairy tale. There is real wisdom at work in our lives. Although she appears repetitive, she is not. Every movement is a new reality. Nature is not a machine but a conscious, intimate, breathing presence that creates and sustains us. We can enter this reality directly if we wish, by slowing our senses down, releasing our attention and waiting....

ENTERING THE DOMAN OF NATURE January 5

Relating to Nature begins with listening.

Go outside and listen to everything around you ... then listen farther and farther away.
Listen as far away as you can.

What happens?

The receptivity to listen beyond the reach of our cultural senses is a vital skill if we wish to relate to Nature as an Intelligence that guides mankind.

A beautiful surprise awaits you.

---

1 Sutherland page 206 COT 2nd edition

KEEPING THE TRUTH — January 6

Keep silent about your experiences until you are aware of who is listening, inside and outside.

Wait until you pass beyond that which you want to relate to others. Then, from the future, look back and speak.

If you speak before your cup is full, there is a loss of relatedness to the Tide. This can create power without love ... you will be lost and alone. You will fail to find peace ... and you may not even know the difference.

Too much talking, too soon, will cause depletion of understanding and leave only word relics. Teaching from ideas, rather than from a living experience, will cause depletion in the soul and discourage students.

REST — January 7

Rest is the foundation of Health.

Rest as much as you do not rest.
Steal time to be alone with the Health.
Be receptive to restoration from Love.

ENDPOINTS AND WHOLENESS — January 8

A traditional Osteopathic treatment ends in wholeness.

In Sutherland's training, with Dr. Still and Dr. Hoover, great emphasis was placed on appreciation of the involuntary motion in the whole at the end of the treatment. Dr. Sutherland trained Dr. Wales and Dr. Day, and they in turned trained me, that the endpoint occurred after the stillpoint when motion returned to the whole of the Fluid Body and was stable. The stability that heralded the endpoint was three cycles of Primary Respiration that were of equal amplitude and tempo.[1]

1 see Notes and Bibliography

WHOLENESS

January 9

Treat the whole patient

Treating the whole patient is often appreciated more as a philosophy than a reality. It is sad that so much of reality is lost in philosophy. The whole is a living reality that can be appreciated directly.

Dr. Still's teaching focuses on something greater than the parts. The parts are effects of the intelligence, power and involuntary motion of the whole. The parts receive their form and physiology from the whole, as well as their fire to do work.

Wholeness can be appreciated directly when the mind is still and neutral, then reality can impress itself upon us. If our observer is active, it keeps us outside of the stillness ... and wholeness is always beyond our reach.

Treating the parts to rebuild the whole is a scientific fallacy. It cannot be done. The function of wholeness is necessary for the development and healing of the parts. Life reaches the parts through the whole. When we sense the whole and it is refreshed ... the parts are realigned and nourished.

PARTS AND THE WHOLE

January 10

Divide your attention between the part and the whole.

The transition into being with the whole arises out of the discipline of divided attention. Each person is a part of the whole of humanity, once this is felt and understood the dimensionality of wholeness changes. If one feels the wholeness of humanity, one becomes less self-centered and enters the movement of the whole. Try this and you will become peaceful.

So it is with a treatment.

The part may be a doorway to the recognition of the Whole, especially if during the entire treatment the attention is divided between the part and the Whole. The attention shifts and the Whole will be in the foreground of one's awareness.... Once the Whole is in the foreground the parts disappear as a reality. Dividing the attention is a constant source of safety and understanding at this level of activity.

During any Osteopathic engagement of the patient the attention is always divided between the object of our attention and a deeper reality... this is true even of direct action methods.

THE CHALLENGE — January 11

You have chosen a life of service.

Your ego will fight for its domain over your heartfelt goal to serve without rewards or goals.... Wholeness is not something the ego can appreciate.

As we move towards an appreciation of wholeness the ego will distract you with seemingly good intentions. Do not listen to its voice. Find the voice of Wholeness and listen deeply. It is a voice of silence.

The voice of the ego cannot create the physical sensation of somatic peace. Only the echo of Wholeness can deepen us and give peace and harmony to our being.

THE ILLUSION — January 12

The parts do not really exist; they are expressions of the whole only.

Knowing this changes the treatment process. When we engage the parts, the only connection we have with Primary Respiration is the effects of transmutation on the parts. When we see the Whole, the therapeutic forces come into view and demonstrate the movement of the Whole, that appears to be in the parts ... but that is only an appearance. The reality is the Whole is moving—not the parts.

THE WHOLENESS OF BEING January 13

Being whole means one does not partition life.

Me ends ... as it does, so do all the contrasts that we engage in as part of the traffic of the culture. All the pieces of life become Life. The flow of the Supreme Intelligence through everything eliminates many prejudices. Conflict ends.

REST January 14

Before you end your day, rest.............then go to bed.

Take your well-being seriously and attend to the foundation of Health—rest.
You are not as alone as you think; when you rest you realize this.

ANATOMY January 15

Anatomy is......................?

Dr. Still was not a structuralist. His vision of what one feels during palpation is quite unique and holistic. In his writings he refers to "descriptive anatomy"[1] as form. Form means something quite different from structure. He describes tissue as "soft parts."[2] The word soft here is very important.

When we can feel anatomy something is lesioned. Normal soma feels like a watery form and the fascial planes are not palpable.

Can you think as to why the anatomy disappears when the "withering fields"[3] are restored?

---

1 Still page 17 Philosophy of Osteopathy
2 A.T. Still Page 17 Philosophy of Osteopathy
3 Still page 39 Philosophy of Osteopathy See Bibliography and Notes

ANATOMY AS FUNCTION — January 16

"I want to impress upon your minds that physiology is as much a part of anatomy as a wing is part of a chicken."[1]

I really enjoy Still's sense of humor and common sense reflected in these words. After hearing his words and letting them settle deeper during palpation, I awakened to a realization: There is no anatomy in the manner in which we think about and teach it.

There are fluid motions and there is form and physiology and they arrive as a singularity in the embryo. This is a subject for long reflection.

ANATOMY AS FUNCTION — January 17

"Remembering that in the room of histology you are still studying anatomy"[2]

Dr. Still takes us into the microscopic as the "machinery that executes every day, hour and minute of life."[3] This is an element of the whole, not a part to be separated during palpation. If dysfunction occurs then this compartment may become separate from the whole and we may feel it, but only because there is disease. Normal function does not reveal the histology as separate place. It is popular to palpate compartments rather than the real wholeness. This places limits on the amount of healing possible.

ANATOMY AS WHOLE — January 18

"It would not be a chicken without every part"[4]

A.T. Still again deflects our rigid minds into the simple truth. The whole is a chicken not the sum of the parts. You and your

1 Still page 17 Philosophy of Osteopathy
2 Still page 17 Philosophy Of Osteopathy
3 Still page 18 Philosophy of Osteopathy
4 Still page 17 Philosophy of Osteopathy

patients are not the parts. Your name is a wholeness. It reflects the beingness of who you are. Do you feel yourself more as whole being or as bunch of parts? So it is with palpation. You listen to the whole, not the parts....

STILL COMMENTS January 19

"The Osteopath reasons, if he reasons at all that order and health are inseparable..."

"And that when order in all parts is found, disease cannot prevail, and if order is complete and disease should be found, there is no use for order. .... order and health are universally one in union."[1]

Dr. Still uses the word 'order' frequently. The modern use of this word could make the meaning appear more shallow than he intended. The word has a very deep origin. It means the perfect work of a Supreme Intelligence.

ANATOMY IS January 20

"What I mean by anatomy ...."

"Form and places ... blood and fluids moving .... Physiology ...production and purification of blood and fluids that... nourish and sustain the whole human body.... Histology... what that machinery ... does [constantly]....Chemistry...the laws of association of substances .... nature ... compounds and combines elements ... Observation and detection of abnormal ... effects ... that cause ... disease.[2]

This summarizes two and one half pages from A.T. Still's

1 Still page 16-19 Philosophy of Osteopathy. See Notes and Bibliography

2 Still page 16-19 Philosophy of Osteopathy. See Notes and Bibliography

Philosophy of Osteopathy. One must see the great mystery of livingness that Still reports and marvel at his skill and knowledge. His legacy is humbling. Our profession is based upon skills that we must reconnect to, as they were lost along the road somewhere.

There is no anatomy in the way we usually think about it. There can be no structure. Transmutation is dynamic.

REST — January 21

Rest.... Rest.... rest ... rest ... until you end.

Rest in your wholeness, without using a technique to get there.
The path is written in you at conception.
This path is a gift to you, so you can get home. It appears when you are naturally neutral.
Do not let your suffering create the path for you, it will not work.

KNOWLEDGE AND UNDERSTANDING — January 22

"A little learning is a dangerous thing; drink deep or taste not the Pierian spring"[1]

These words, from Alexander Pope's essay "On Criticism," were used by Dr. Sutherland as an opening to the first edition of Osteopathy in the Cranial Field. The essay is long, I would suggest that you read it; it gives a clear picture of how critics generally have no understanding of the topic they are criticizing.

Sutherland was criticized heavily. He weathered the storm with compassion. Once when a colleague left his program to pursue their personal understanding, many people chastised

1 Alexander Pope (1688 1744). An Essay on Criticism, 1709. See also Bibliography and Notes

that person. But, Sutherland's response was: "there is foam on the surface of the sea, the wind will come and disperse it." His understanding of Primary Respiration was not from books or imitation of technique, he was a student of the Tide and he lived the consequences ... in this case compassion and trust, rather than judgement and anger. If we do not understand compassion from the Tide itself, we can become possessive of our one point of view and create divisions amongst our fellow Osteopaths.

Later, Dr. Becker helped me immensely. While in a board meeting for the S.C.T.F., people began to fight and yell harshly. Rollin was sitting next to me; I was in shock at what I saw happening. I leaned over and whispered "Rollin! Where is the Tide? Why are they acting like this? He said, "wait ten years it will heal." He was not being sarcastic; he meant it and in his voice I heard compassion and patience ... it impressed me. He had understanding that would not acutely polarize his heart.

A little knowledge creates projection....
Knowledge from the Tide creates love.

THE TRANSITION

January 23

Knowledge begins with our education.

Later, as the Tide heals us, we come to know being loved beyond our belief. All our knowledge will die in the movement of this healing in ourselves.

Knowledge in the western world is a commodity; it can lead to a sense of power and superiority. This illusion can destroy a profession and certainly institutions.

Knowledge in the ancient traditions is an effect of communion with the Divine. There is direct knowledge from the Tide that comes with us at conception and stays with us throughout life. Osteopathy is from and about that knowledge.

Pride is not as easy to unveil in oneself as one might think ...

Pride is deceptive. However, it can be discovered by the effect it has on one's neutrality.

Early in my time with Ruby she saw my pride very clearly. She said she could not take me any deeper until I changed. I still met with her every two weeks. She would sit in her rocking chair and tell stories about her grandson. I was bored and wanted more lessons ... more knowledge. She waited. I firmly believed that God had given me more sensitivity than her. In my morning meditations I tried to be humble. But the darkness prevailed. I loved her and to be trapped in feeling superior to her was painful ... very painful. I struggled. No result. Though I did not know this at the time, I was using pride to fight pride and making it all the stronger.

Every visit to her home, as I knocked, her sweet voice could be heard through the closed door. "Are you perfect yet?" she would say in a warm manner. I was so frustrated with my incapacity for change that I was getting anxious. This went on for months and months ... no new lessons, just boring stories and then I would leave and go home.

Finally, I caved in. Ruby, I said, "I cannot do it. I am powerless to overcome this pride in myself. As much as I love you, I am harboring a superiority complex."

Of course she knew this, and I knew she knew it, and we both knew we were working on it. I was ready to quit because I could not loosen the grip of the desire for knowledge for the sake of power. It was disguised, of course, as a desire to help my patients. The pride wanted to be seen as the healer.

She saw my sincerity and restarted the lessons. I was humbled by her action. Now I listened to her more easily. I was not grasping so hard or resting on the laurels of the Tide's work in the patients, thinking I was the skill. It took years and much help from the Tide but I am slowly becoming more whole.

Humility does not compare ... this alone is key for those

interested in the hidden inside of themselves. It is neutral. If your neutral is steady and you feel it, it will not be long before you can tell pride by the loss of inner peace and neutrality.

THE NEW LANDSCAPE

January 25

The persona of the Tide Loves without cause.

The Tide does not love the best and dislike the worst. It does not admire our knowledge or skill. It does not wait for the physician to prove worthy. It waits for a doorway and then presents itself to the physician, clothed as something familiar, in order to allow the patient to receive help.

It humbles itself, because we are not able to be humble ourselves.

THE HEALTH

January 26

At the edge of one's boundary is the Health.

Go to meet it.
How?
Love something with innocence
one thing... and it will open a door that you closed.

LIFE IS WHOLENESS January 27

Life is wholeness.

It is a mystery beyond our potential to understand. We must consider becoming comfortable with our ignorance, becoming a living organism in "The Sea Around Us"[1], nurtured and loved through an indwelling sense of direction. We move beyond being complete, content or fulfilled … into the Holy River of Life.

REST January 28

Rest is a time of Return.

Rest is a time of Return. One goes Home to the Health. There is a very strong movement in all of us towards normal. This indwelling flow is the direction of ease … but we rarely are neutral enough, for long enough, to allow the transmutations to occur which carry us ashore to safety.

The following meditation imitates Mother's Natures quest for normal.

One can sit or lay down but the body must be at ease, that is to say, as neutral as possible. Remember that Osteopathic principles state that there is an Indwelling Therapeutic Process; in this meditation you will see that principle at work. There are three aspects to be appreciated:
The Health expressing Itself, the shifts in thoracic respiration, and the movement of the observer.

Let the Health express Itself.

This part of the meditation is noticing what is already at work…the Health expressing Itself. Seen or unseen, the Health is fully present and in motion. But how and where ones sees

---

1 Sutherland page 255, 300 Contributions of Thought see also Bibliography and Notes

this is highly variable so, as Emily Dickinson wrote "not knowing when the dawn will come I open every door...."[1] Her words are so true. A word of caution: do not try and open up to it or give it space. Simply see the Health as it is.

Notice the activity of Thoracic Respiration.

The breathing - just watch and you will see it 'head for home'. It will do direct, indirect, and opposing physiological motion. It will slow, speed up, pause, and occasionally end. As it ends there is another breath - not the Tide, as we know it - but the Master breathing. This breath comes up the center and is a nutritive liquid light ... it creates many changes ... you will understand ownership of the house in a new manner. You will be suffused with being and serenity that is LOVE incarnate.

The location of the fulcrum of the breathing may be more superficial and anterior, that is to say towards the world around you or it may be deep behind the midline near the meeting place. This will be self-evident as you do the exercise, so do not let my language confuse you.

The observer is the seer

The observer—where is it? Outside? In front of the breathing? In the breathing? Behind the breathing? Or has it reconnected with the true self? Watch ... it will shift, and as this happens, like a blending, your beingness will change towards a glorious neutral....

METHODOLOGY — January 29

Look for something you've never seen before.

The difficulty with being original is that we have habits. Our habits and method of treatment veil any possible awareness of the therapeutic process of the Tide.

Dr. Sutherland's methodology began confrontationally; he

1 Emily Dickinson Complete Poems 1924. Part Two: Nature

used force to communicate with the Mechanism. This only created chaos and was dangerous. His writing shows he almost killed himself in this process. Later, he tried to "get as far as one can from the physical sense"[1]

Sutherland's methods changed because he was constantly working to develop a relationship with the Mechanism. Over time these efforts and his sincere willingness allowed him to shift his perspective and his methodology.

Clear observation of new material requires that one look for something one has never seen before. This is not easy. Try this when you walk outside your home. There is the familiar, but what do you notice when you look for something new, something you've never appreciated before.

Try this at the end of a treatment when you are just observing.

STUDY — January 30

Dr. Sutherland was not afraid to be awed by the obvious, even when he doubted what he saw.

He started to see articular motion of the boney cranium in adults. He consulted experts and they told him with certainty that the cranial bones were fused in the adults. Therefore he doubted that there could be motion and set out to prove just that.

He then did a very interesting thing. He took a pen knife and dissected along the sutures of the temporal bone. He was able to dissect out the bone along sutures in an adult. The boney articulations were then seen directly. If there is a joint then there is no fusion. The experts still rambled about the fusion, even though he dissected a single cranial bone from an adult skull. His interest in cranial motion was peaked. He chose to "dig" on.[2]

1 Sutherland page 210 Contributions of Thought
2 Sutherland See Bibliography and Notes

Reread the first few chapters of The Teachings in The Science of Osteopathy. Study his attitude and you will see how this profession is scientific.

In the late eighties, Eliot Blackman, D.O. and I spoke privately many times about sensing a dural structure between the middle and anterior cranial fossa. Magoun showed nothing of this in his writing. Finally, we were given the opportunity to direct a dissection looking at the region between the middle and anterior cranial fossa. We were astounded at what we found, as was the professor, Dr. Willard. There was a thickened dural band - at least 5 times thicker than the falx or the tent. Now, almost twenty years later, and many dissections to validate this fact, there are still some who say it is useless information. Be that as it may, there are many thousands of children who have been helped by this knowledge in clinics all over the world.

These facts were first discovered by listening to the natural motion of life in tissue. Sutherland and Still were explorers. They did not rely on theories, but sought and relied on knowledge gained through direct contact with patients and natural law. It is our legacy to follow new terrain as it appears.

You have discovered something new yourself....but you may not know it because you let it pass by your awareness.... I am sure we are all seeing new landscapes ... some may challenge the status quo.

All the more reason to look again with respect.

STUDY — January 31

Sharing with a group of fellow travelers is what grows this profession.

It is what sustains the Truth that slowly unveils itself from generation to generation. The older Osteopaths love to see the younger take the reins and ride ahead.

THE SENSES AND THE INSTINCT February 1

The senses have many connections.

The five senses have been discussed by Mystics for thousands of years. The Greek Mystics studied the senses in detail. Aristotle first named them.

In spiritual literature, the idea is often presented that the senses are fraught with worldly attachment. I disagree. Osteopathy has several truths that prove that the senses have a deep relation with the Health.

Before we follow this further, have you noticed the difference between the instinctual and the rational minds? How are the senses operating in each case? Can you direct the senses to be in either place or is it random?

Instinct is not learned behavior. Instinct is a God given interface with the movements of nature. We are designed to know the weather, to feel danger pre-cognitively and be still, to see and listen to the horizon, to know where our friends are even at great distances, to smell at great distances, to have an instinctual sense of reverence for Life, to give thanks when we survive a storm, to seek silence as a resting place. Instinct has a heart that listens for guidance.

Most of these functions are hidden in the cellar of our consciousness having been imprisoned there by our education and modern conveniences.

Seek out the instinct and listen to its voice. Then you may find the deeper landscapes of the senses. Being in the wild opens this world.

THE INNER SENSES February 2

We have inner senses and outer senses.

The inner senses have been suppressed. The inner sense of smell is the intuitive understanding of a moment. The inner sense of taste is to have a conscience. The inner sense of sight is a vision, a lucid dream. The inner sense of hearing is listening to the pauses. The inner sense of touch is to be touched by the flow of love. These inner senses operate at a deeper and more integrated level than the cultured senses. As a matter of fact, the two kinds of senses are often in contradiction. This can lead to continued ambivalence about life and immune depletion.

To hear the inner senses the rational mind must be quiet.
We must pause to hear them.

THE ORIGINAL SENSES February 3

"I love my fellow man because I see God in his face and his form."[1]

At eighty-six, Dr. Still expressed a very deep and abiding Osteopathic truth. He reported seeing the Divine Image in man. This vision is usually reserved for mystics who have contemplated for long and arduous years. Seeing the Health in others, their Divinity, occurs when the physician's senses are aware of Health. We begin with small glimpses of this possibility. It matures as the Health touches us.

REST February 4

True rest is being in the presence of the Beloved.

Find a room inside the Health where you are a guest in the Master's House. Here one gives up the illusion of ownership ... even of breathing. Sutherland points us here when he talks about being closer to the Creator than your own breath.

1 Still, published on a reproduction of a photograph of Still, which is in some editions of the Autobiography

BEING CENTERED BY DEITY February 5

In his 1965 Sutherland Memorial Lecture Dr. Becker mentions 'being centered by Deity.'[1] The experience of this is not automatic; one must notice the presence of a principle that centers oneself and feel the love that binds everyone to the Health. One's seeing, hearing, smelling, touching, and tasting are all reversed. Instead of seeing one feels seen, instead of touching one feels touched ....

The senses unite into One Sense and then....

THE LESION February 6

A lesion is an attempt by the Whole to isolate stress in a part of the organism to prevent lesioning of the whole.

THE LESION FIELD February 7

A lesion field is not between bones; it has a form and boundaries that contain all elements of the patient. The boundaries of a lesion field pass through bones, tissues, viscera, fluid fields, psyche... The penetrating forces of the lesion field make a design not limited by the biomechanics of the soma.

THE FORCE VECTORS February 8

The force vectors are geometrically precise and are gathered upon a fulcrum like the strings of a parachute. The fulcrum is there first.

1 Becker page 25 Life in Motion, see also Bibliography and Notes

THE FULCRUM

February 9

Dr. Fulford opened my eyes and mind when he said to me: "The fulcrum is established pre-cognitively by the Tide before the impact of the insult."[1] The Tide sees the future and establishes a fulcrum through which it channels the forces of the trauma.

THE TIMING

February 10

Dr. Alan Becker studied lesions and their natural progress. He found that 36 and one half hours before the symptoms appear there is a shock that sets the system up to lesion. He was quite insistent that in taking the patient's history we should pursue the cause that made the system lesion. I have done this for twenty-five years and the tracking of the history in detail can bring insight that can cure. Try and pin-down the exact moment the symptoms appeared, then track the history to exactly thirty-six and one-half hours prior. Once you have reached that point the patient may not remember anything that seems important - just wait and let them ponder. Things will be recalled.

REST

February 11

Dr. Sutherland and most Osteopaths have seen rest as a vital part of the healing process. Today it is definitely overlooked. One needs to study rest and what happens inside the organism at rest. Dr. Sutherland recommended the book called A Philosophy Of Rest by Ella Adelia Fletcher. This text is still available at www.kessinger.com. Please read this.

1 See Bibliography and Notes

IATROGENIC LESIONS February 12

Because of Alan Becker's discoveries I have found that if I make a mistake, and over treat or add inappropriate force, a simple rebalancing will erase these anomalies and the treatment can continue. The lesion created by the operator does not become fixed in the body system for many hours so reversal is very simple. Alan helped me appreciate this and treat accordingly. Fresh injuries can be treated more easily than one might think, if one has this understanding.

Simply go to the fulcrum of the fresh lesion and find the stillness in it. Sense the whole and wait.

THE WHOLE February 13

The Whole lesions.

The Health organizes the lesioning parts, their shape and fulcrum. Lesions are not stupid, their I.Q. is very high. Lesions are connected directly to the Health by motion present.

FINDING CAUSE February 14

The fulcrum in the lesion field is a doorway.

Through this doorway one reaches the next level of cause.

FINDING CAUSE February 15

An Osteopath does not think on the shallow ground of the Allopathic model.

Why did the patient get sick?

FINDING CAUSE

February 16

The Cause of an illness is not the illness itself but how one became susceptible.

FINDING CAUSE

February 17

The doorway through the fulcrum in the lesion field of the chief complaint leads to another lesion field with boundaries and force vectors and a fulcrum. Follow this trail until the Tide stops the passage. Here is where you begin treatment—not in the area of the chief complaint. If this sounds strange to you, then you must consider how you think and why. Osteopathy is not physiotherapy or orthopedics. Nor is it a structural science. It is a precise movement through cause … into Cause, both in the relative and the absolute sense. The cause of an illness can be easily overlooked in the history and the evaluation— When you are intent on finding the Cause … you will not be distracted by superficial interpretations.

REST

February 18

Go to bed 2 hours early.

FINDING CAUSE February 19

A patient comes in with x-rays, the symptoms of cervical stenosis and surgical expectation. All the basic diagnostics lead to the cervical stenosis. Severe unrelenting pain in the lower cervicals, insomnia, swollen hands with loss of grip strength and situational depression. This has been acute for several months. Nothing has helped. She is a surgical candidate. One could easily settle into the treatment of this severe case with intent of treatment of the stenosis.

We are trained to look for cause.

Once the cervical lesion field is delineated and the fulcrum is found around C6, one continues through the fulcrum as a doorway. This is not following myofascial continuity but following the force vectors. The doorway leads to another 'place', the thoraco-lumbar juncture. Here is another lesion field that feels like it made the chronic stenosis acute. But, one moves into the fulcrum and passes through into another room. This lesion field covers most of the patient, it is old. It is an emotional trauma from long ago.

Which lesion is using up the most power?

One continues to go deeper until the Tide stops the progress and says, "treat here." One neglects the obvious and goes to cause. Over two treatments the patient gets sixty-percent better. After two more treatments the patient is ninety percent better. How is that possible? How many illnesses has this one lesion caused?

Think and ask questions.

CAUSE February 20

There are relative and absolute causes.

In his 1965 Sutherland Memorial Lecture, Dr. Becker wrote beautifully about Absolute Cause. Again we must think like Osteopaths not "cause-and-effect" Allopaths. Think about this for yourself as you read Dr. Becker's words.

CAUSE AND THE HEALTH — February 21

The Health creates the lesion to protect the whole in an act of wisdom.

When we hate lesions in ourselves, we miss the real story of love. Does hating a lesion help healing? Self-pity is a poison. Feeling healthy or ill is the same fulcrum. Neutrality can improve both levels of function. How often do you consult with your patients on this?

MIND, MOTION, MATTER — February 22

The basis of Osteopathy lies in these words.

The Mind Dr. Still speaks of, is not the academic mind or the rational, but the Mind of Creation—the Supreme Intelligence. This Divine breathes Life, as it does animation occurs. The Breath of Life moves into the material, creates form, and spiritualizes Matter.

There is a Great Mystery creating the metabolic Motion from which all forms emerge as a Wholeness. A deep study of embryology would show this picture to be accurate.

MOTION — February 23

"Life is that calm force sent forth by Deity to vivify all nature."[1]

All of life, everything that seems well or ill … every motion you can perceive with any sense … is Life. People running, the door closing, the lesion field, the Health … everything is ultimately moved by that slow vivifying force. One motion is all there is in the whole.

1 Still, page 101 Philosophy and Mechanical Principles

MATTER February 24

The ancient writings in Sanskrit, the ancient Greek thinkers, the modern sciences all use the idea that we have materiality. The problem is that it is not static, but dynamic. It is not segmented, but whole. In the human being, matter is not inert. Spirit, matter, and all categories of energy are being renewed and dying so fast that one can miss the singularity of life. To divide our sensory experience into compartments can lead to false conclusions. Matter is as busy as spirit.

REST February 25

Homeostasis and rest are related.

Homeostasis is the perfect point of physiological neutrality

DIVISIONS February 26

In the cranial work we study tissue, fluid, and the fluid in the fluid. In fact these compartments only exist in unresolved lesion fields. If we separate these levels when we treat we can slow the healing process or lesion the patient. These categories only have meaning during diagnosis. Life co-mingles and transmutates so nothing can stay in a compartment. Everything changes its nature constantly. This is why growth and healing are so amazing.

DIVISIONS February 27

Rates and zones are learning tools and helpful in diagnostics.

Once the organism is in a dynamic neutral all divisions end. They cannot be found. Sometimes this is a bit of a surprise.

THE ENDING February 28

The ending of partitions occurs as we heal.

We feel undifferentiated and transparent to the Breath of Life. We no longer feel ourselves or others but all is one ... and nothing.

THE SPACE BETWEEN March 1

"'Tis the mortar in the Space between the bricks that holds the structure together"[1]

Sutherland is pointing us away from the known and from the structural addiction that we all have. He is moving us towards recognizing Creative movement through everything. Sutherland repeats this important concept saying, "read the space between the physiological centers within the fourth ventricle." [2]These quotes tell us that focusing on structure is not as engaging as focusing on the space between our images. Sutherland points our focus towards something, which he calls, endless Space. He has left structure and function behind as he ascends towards Cause. There are parallels here to Dr. Schooley's article in the 1953 OCA Journal "The Fulcrum."

In the development of any function/structure the space is first defined as an opening of the pattern in the fluid. Space opens ... function moves in. This truth can effect how our treatments are oriented to the Tide.

1 Sutherland page 254 2nd edition Contributions of Thought
2 Sutherland page 254 2nd edition Contributions of Thought

THE SPACE BETWEEN March 2

"The space between atoms is pure Intelligent energy .... the fulcrum of all matter and its function permeates all the space of the Infinite universe." [1]

The space between becomes the center point of one's attention. In the 1953 OCA Journal Dr. Schooley capitalizes the words Intelligence and Infinite to point us towards the Divine mystery that is indwelling.

Dr. Still said, " Life is a sub-stance which fills all of the space of the whole universe."[2] The word Life was a reference to the wholeness of creation and its presence in between what appears as matter.

If we follow this through when we enter the space between, the anatomy is veiled. One finds a sense of space and ... Creation. Enter the seams between the anatomy and you will be in Space.

Work to sense Space without feeling anatomy. What happens is quite remarkable.

THE EMBRYONIC SAC March 3

This commentary will seem like metaphor and yet as the years melt, you may realize that metaphor is a part of our oral tradition and as such is more of a living reality than not.

The embryonic sac as an internal reality within oneself plays a dramatic role in educating one to the indwelling spirit of the Divine Health in everyone. Within this sac we find a soft golden light and the form of an embryo. Interestingly, the shape of the embryo only takes up half the space, as if there is room for another presence.

---

1 Dr. Schooley, The Fulcrum, OCA 1953 Journal
2 Still page 279 Research and Practice

REST — March 4

Let the known disappear.

The thoughts and emotions may flow a little; be at peace with human nature and do not despair. Rest in not knowing.

THE LESIONED FLUID BODY — March 5

The idea of a Fluid Body lesioning is a major insight of William Garner Sutherland. Read his writings, especially after 1948, as his sense of the fluid changes.

The Health creates the Fluid Body. It has a specific form and three kinds of fluctuations that hold the form. The Fluid Body can lesion and when it does it creates many phenomena including somatic dysfunction. One could reflect on somatic dysfunction as "fluid" phenomena.

PRIMARY RESPIRATION — March 6

The distinction is made between Primary Respiration and the effects of Primary Respiration to promote a clear understanding of what it means to follow the intention of Primary Respiration. What do you think is the difference between Primary Respiration and the effects of Primary Respiration? Is the Breath of Life different from both?

VOID — March 7

Before we arrive into the world beyond rates, we enter a void.

In the void we are alone with our ego.... Our response to this isolation determines what happens next.

THE PLACE BEYOND RATES — March 8

As one moves from place to place, following the fulcrum, we arrive at levels of activity where there are no inhalation nor exhalation periods. The living process is balanced. There is space, Dynamic Stillness, Presence, the movement of Creation ... along with the physical sensation of eternity and love.

BALANCED TENSION — March 9

The balance point and the point of balance are different.

Think on this.

BALANCED LIGAMENTOUS TENSION — March 10

The balance point is reached ...

The balance point is reached through motion testing and the direction of ease. The balance point then holds us, quietly, until the potency enters and begins a therapeutic event. Using this technique, relying on the Health, one finds the results are more lasting and profound.

REST — March 11

Do not believe you have rested, ever.

Begin again and seek eternity

BALANCED MEMBRANOUS TENSION March 12

The Technique of Balanced Ligamentous Tension, applied to the Dural Membranes, is called Balanced Membranous Tension. Make sure you know how much force or ease is being engaged when you work. Motion testing and barrier have been eliminated in the principles of the Biodynamic model. Diagnostics have not. Know the limitations of your palpatory skills in diagnosis and therapeutics. When you engage motion testing and barrier you have passed your limit. Stay inside the ease and let the neutral evolve.

BALANCED MEMBRANOUS TENSION March 13

Sutherland preferred indirect methods, the direction of ease. Read the Cranial Manual by the Lippincotts. The balance point is a suspension of all tensions around a point of balance. Can you feel this: the balance point in the tissue and the point of balance in the whole area?

This leads to the direct awareness of Transmutation. Tissue becomes fluid ….

NO DURA ON THE BONES March 14

There is no reason why anyone should want to manipulate the Dura Mater to move the bones. The Dura Mater is not without intrinsic sensibilities. To apply force to this tissue shows a lack of understanding of its physiology and the anatomy of the meninges. The bones have their own membranes, called the outer and inner periosteum, which are metabolically active in managing osteoblastic and osteoclastic activity, as well as in shaping the bones. The envelopes around the cranial bones are not the Dura mater. Anne Wales told us that Dr. Sutherland said many times that people want to move the bones rather than the envelopes they were in.

A review of the development of the ectomeninx would be helpful in restoring an understanding of function. The word meninx or meninges comes from Greek, and it means the coverings of the brain; it does not just refer to the Dura Mater. Herein lies a contrast between embryology and gross anatomical terms.

The histology of different meninges has been veiled by the gross anatomy resulting in a lack of understanding of function.

There is no anatomy like one sees in dissection!

NO MOTION TESTING March 15

Intrinsic to every lesion is healthy motion, what we call Motion Present.

It is a thread that connects to the Health. Watch the lesion field for movement. Smallest does not mean weakest.

THORACIC RESPIRATION March 16

Thoracic Respiration as it occurs in the Health is fire of equal magnitude to Primary Respiration. They are one in essence and origin.

This is so important to appreciate in the treatment of children.

ONENESS March 17

In the Biodynamic Model of Primary Respiration Oneness represents the union of the soul, the spirit and the breathing. Thoracic and Primary Respiration are one. Oneness is a marriage of the soul (our being) to the spirit (our Health)

resulting in something

that contains

neither.

REST March 18

One is much relieved.

ONENESS March 19

All reciprocal tensions are given up into the Breath of Life; peace and harmony suspend a sense of collective being.

ONENESS March 20

The True Midline stands in eternity, it has never moved in time;

It cannot walk from one place to another as we do.

ONENESS March 21

The individual enters all of humanity as a sense of self.

ONENESS March 22

Perception is transparent.

HEALING March 23

Healing is the emergence of Originality.

OSTEOPATHY March 24

Disease is the process of getting well.

REST March 25

If you don't rest you'll pay for it.

EVOLUTION March 26

We evolve in our skill not through removing lesions, but by what we learn at the endpoints.

EVOLUTION March 27

Creation and evolution are not at odds.

Evolution is the overcoming of the barriers in oneself so that one may feel the movement of Creation and continue to grow under the influence of the Health.

CREATION/EVOLUTION March 28

Evolution is self-fulfilling.

It occurs in time. Creation is self-emptying. It is Eternity.

CREATION March 29

The movement of creation never ended. It is here now.

CREATION March 30

There is no rate in self-emptying

SILENCE March 31

The following was collected from an unknown source.

Participants in the courses added the rest. Each one was reviewed by a number of elders for authenticity.

Silence vibrating is Creation
Silence flowing is Love
Silence shared is Friendship

Silence seen is Infinity
Silence heard is Adorable
Silence muted is Fear

Silence expressed is Beauty
Silence maintained is Strength
Silence omitted is Suffering

Silence Deified is Bliss

Silence allowed is Rest
Silence recorded is Scripture
Silence preserved is our Tradition

Silence given is Initiating
Silence received is Joy
Silence perceived is Knowledge

Silence stabilized is Fulfillment
Silence illuminated is Vision

Silence touched is Spiritual Growth
Silence shaped is Form
Embraced by Silence is Grace

Silence treasured is endless Readiness
Silence heard answering is Knowing
Silence breathing is Recognition

Silence remembered is Home
Silence embraced is limitless Possibilities
Silence surrender to is Guidance

Silence completed is Oneness
Silence to begin is Freedom
Silence experienced, Is
Silence ripened is Incarnation
Silence lived is Normal

REST April 1

Repose means to rest in the arms of the Beloved.

One sleeps in a special way, without tomorrow or today. It is as if one needed to rest forever.

SILENCE AND STILLNESS April 2

Silence is the garden, Stillness is the rain.

Silence is the word incarnating.
Stillness is the action of transmutation.
One notices the difference in many ways.

EFFORT April 3

The effort to be active or passive is achieved through will; it can only lead you to engaging an effect of the Tide.

The true source of doing or effort must be the Tide. Be neutral, the Tide will pass through you. Then the intention of the Tide becomes what you are expressing.

EFFORT April 4

Do not be a diagnostician at home, leave it at work.

Our skills need to be used only for service.
Labeling others who have not asked for our help is unethical

EFFORT April 5

It is popular to tell students to back off when using too much force.

This accomplishes no education. Give the student something constructive to do.... like look for a different landscape or therapeutic force. Learning takes many years.
Backing off is not a real place to go to.

EFFORT April 6

Is there a deeper therapeutic process than the one I am engaging?

Even when the therapeutics are going well look for a deeper process. This will lead to a surprise in most cases—even in the experts.

EFFORT April 7

How much willpower?

Very little, or none. Measuring your willpower is fun. It is very subtle. Try this, a story I got from a Steiner teacher.
Sit down in the garden next to a carrot. Wait until you are centered, then compare your willpower or effort to the effort of the carrot. As silly as this sounds it really helped me see how intense I was.

REST April 8

As one approaches neutrality there is a sense of stillness in the landscape where one is sitting.

It suspends us in a more complete sense of Life.

EFFORT
April 9

Listen to nothing, shut the senses off.

The nothingness is something.

STILLNESS
April 10

There are stillpoints through which transmutation occurs.

To know this phenomena one must see the activity of the stillness. The first level does not promote transmutation, yet third level does, in a deep manner.

TRANSMUTATION
April 11

Sutherland like Still chose his words carefully and fully.

Today, words are used very loosely and out of context. Transmutation was used by Ovid in the text Metamorphosis. It means the change of state of one thing into a completely different state. It implies alchemical change. Changes of being that, if seen, would appear miraculous. One can see transmutation when the Tide directs its potency into a static lesion field. It enters the lesion and then the lesion is gone. No process is visible, as one would see with transformation. It just happens in a magical way.

Watch for this phenomena. At first you may not believe your eyes. As Sutherland said, it is "uncanny."[1]

---

1 Sutherland Page 166 Teachings in the Science of Osteopathy

TRANSMUTATION April 12

I wonder how many people actually think about what this word means.

We all want to understand the process, or to see the process, or to grasp the process.Do not analyze while treating and you will see this word in action.

TRANSMUTATION April 13

Faith in the Tide will prove what Primary Respiration is.

Just having words means nothing. We are too dependent on ideologies. We are too dependent on our interest in our personal psychology to see the option of change without finding the cause. Treat as if your faith is real and see what happens. Faith as an experiment may prove something.

TRANSMUTATION April 14

Tissue expressing neutral becomes a gel without fascial planes.

REST April 15

Rest occurs in time. Repose in eternity.

TRANSMUTATION April 16

Healing occurs without a time frame.

Here now, then gone. Do not call the lesion back into being out of self-interest ... accept Love as a reality.

TRANSMUTATION April 17

During the inhalation period of Primary Respiration the sphenoid becomes transparent and one sees liquid light.

We cannot see these things unless we are centered by the Tide and are aware of It as our Cause. The tissue under the influence of transmutation becomes more and more fluid and transparent.

TRANSUBSTANTIATION April 18

Another old word.

The miraculous enters time. The simple becomes eternal.
Transformation: direct or indirect action.
Transmutation: no action from operator; natural laws at work.
Transubstantiation: Divine intervention.

AUGMENTATION April 19

Augmentation was incorporated by Sutherland into the therapeutic process.

The most basic form was used to assist in creating a neutral in tissue that was being engaged using Balanced Membranous Tension. The tissue was taken indirectly into ease and carried in that direction until inertia presented itself. At this point, instead of adding force himself, he had the patient cooperate in a manner that would cause the tissue to continue towards a neutral state. For example, if an A-O lesion was to be released, he would start in the direction of ease. Once there was resistance to ease, he would have the patient move a foot, in flexion or extension, to support further ease and movement towards neutral. The choice of positional augmentation was based upon the response in the A-O tissues. The foot is a long way from the lesion site. Sutherland liked long levers and said, as reported by both Anne Wales and Ruby Day "the longer the lever the greater the therapeutic power."[1] As the tissues went to neutral with this assistance, the Tide came into the field and transmutated the lesion

Try this principle. It is a wonderful tool and skill builder.

AUGMENTATION April 20

Sutherland also used the patient's control of their breath to initiate augmentation.

As the tissue became neutral and the Tide came into the lesion field, he would ask the patient to breathe in an exaggerated manner. This would augment the direction and force the Tide was introducing into the neutral. Try this: While releasing a rib lesion, neutral is met ... wait ... the Tide comes in to the neutral and begins to compress the Fluid. If the patient is low in vitality ask the patient to breathe out and hold the breath as long as possible or until there is a sense of the synchronization between the Tide and Thoracic Respiration.

1 See Bibliography and Notes

You may sense a crescendo, transmutation of tissue to fluid, and suspension in the Sea Around Us.

Use this tool and see what new understanding of augmentation occurs.

AUGMENTATION April 21

The addition of Thoracic Respiration to the interface of the Tide and the tissue neutral can be done with inhalation, exhalation, or step breathing. The inhalation can be deepened or held; exhalation is the same. Step breathing is a nasal breathing that steps from shallow to full and is stopped at the point where it augments the Tide's establishment of Neutral.

Explore this ... it is an essential feature of Primary and Thoracic Respiration and their mutual fulcrum.

REST April 22

Rest...................................

As you rest, watch your breathing and the breathing of the Sea; there will be great changes if you rest from your observer.

SPONTANEOUS AUGMENTATION April 23

You will notice that in patients with good vitality, and especially in children, that Thoracic Respiration augments the crescendo of the Tidal transmutative efforts.

Often, as the Tide begins the transmutation of the lesion's inertia, and there is a sense of EV4 spreading outwards ... here in this moment, the Thoracic Respiration spontaneously meets the Tide as a single force. The patient deeply sighs, just at the right moment, and then there is a dramatic increase in the release and transmutation. Sutherland called this a "groundswell"[1] referring to the lesion as a little boat on the Sea.

Watch children carefully and you will often see this as an endpoint.

NATURAL AUGMENTATION April 24

Normal function is an expression of natural augmentation.

One of the means we use to determine normal in any single function is whether or not there is augmentation with other functions. For example, with a cerebral vascular accident the insult, if focal, causes the fluid field in the affected area to shrink and compress. There is no effect on the dural or periosteal functions except a minimal loss of vitality. However, the synchronicity between these functions is lost; the result is that they have different rates and expression. This is a loss of natural augmentation. Normally these functions support each other's physiological momentum as an expression of the whole. Sutherland noted this indirectly when he said, "when all the fulcrums are synchronized there will be peace and harmony."[2]

Looking for the presence of natural augmentation is very useful, when you want to look at the refinement in any function.

1 Sutherland Teachings in the Science of Osteopathy see Bibliography and Notes
2 See Bibliography and Notes

INTERNAL AUGMENTATION April 25

Within each lesioned function, it is always true that the tissue, the fluid, and the fluid in the fluid (potency) become independent of each other and take on a limited relationship with the Sea Around Us.

When we are looking at the function of any area of insult we must look at what the elementals are doing. Is there an involuntary motion in each element and are they working together as augmentative principles, or not?
Are the tissue, the fluid, and the fluid within the fluid, on the same fulcrum. Are they moving together? If so you cannot feel these as separate functions. In concussion with memory loss, this is an essential diagnostic tool.

Normal has no visible parts, augmentation is inherently veiled by wholeness.

THE FLUID April 26

This word is a symbol.

It has many deep meanings. It is not water. It is not cerebro-spinal fluid. Sutherland discovered many phenomena related to the fluid. There are many fluids. The ones we think about most are protoplasm, the Fluid Body, and the Health.

The basis of life is protoplasm. Protoplasm is the first moldable substance that can hold an image. This substance is very remarkable. It can become anything. An eye, bile, bone, cerebro-spinal fluid. It is neutral in nature but can be transmutated into any function or form. It is poorly understood by science and currently the definition of protoplasm is being broadened to make it more in line with what is popular in medical thinking. How can it be so diversifiable? It simply is a mystery.

Think about this one substance that becomes everything that is in us, including your mind. This is the essential fluid of life.

THE FLUID BODY April 27

We have coined the term, Fluid Body to symbolize the activity of the fluid as a whole.

It is also called Zone B to differentiate from Zone A, which is tissue that cannot go to Neutral. When we are in perfect Health, the Fluid Body does not exist because then we feel the perfect Fluid Body ... we call this the Health. It has a different transparency than Zone B. Zone B is optically homogenous and silvery-gray. The Health is more transparent and has a quality of liquid light ... like warm honey.

But we must remember that the fluid body can lesion. And as such is different from the Fluid Body of the Health, thusly we have two fluid bodies, one perfect and one that can lesion. The one that can lesion is an intelligent compensatory mechanism to offset the modifying influences of the genetic field.

STILLNESS AND SILENCE April 28

The potency of the stillness is different at different rates. The potency of the Silence is always the same.

REST April 29

Codependency and rest are opposite.

THE PERFECT FLUID BODY April 30

This is the Health.

It can become anything. It is totally transmutable. When we sense this we are on holy ground, outside the laws framed by mankind.

DYING May 1

Dying is what keeps us alive.

Lesions refuse to die and be transformed. Growth occurs when the old dies and the new arises. There is no structure, only form arising and dying.

DEATH AND OSTEOPATHY May 2

There is no death.

Any general practitioner will tell you there is life after death. I was definitely not prepared for the events that occur around the common belief that we end at death. My patients over and over reported events and allowed me be a witness with them as they died. If you have worked with the Tide and someone is dying it is not a negative event that ends with the mindset we often fear. Dr. Still was clear that we live on, he wrote "man is eternal…." [1] How does this strike you?

At death we transpire into the Health.

Access your fear of death and that of your patients … it is a primary lesion.
Helping people transition is part of our responsibility as physicians.

1 Still page 258 Philosophy and Principles of Osteopathy

ZONE C May 3

Zone C is a term that symbolizes the spiritual nature of Primary Respiration.

All of my mentors were aware of a Divine Mystery enshrined in the motions of Primary Respiration. Our relationship, in serving that reality, is Zone C. Dr. Becker in the 1965, Sutherland Memorial Lecture focused on this relationship. He said, "The Deity centers us…." [1]These words need constant vigilance. We do not center ourselves but rather realize the dependency on the Tide to transmutate our awareness.

ZONE C May 4

Dr. Sutherland called the Tide 'Dad.'

There is a persona to the Tide, it is not a biological force. In this persona it is a teacher and a beloved.

It will touch you with love so specific to your need that you will know the words of our mentors are true.

ZONE C May 5

If you are alert and free your request will be met, immediately, in a manner that will heal and inform you of another level of dependency. The spiritual nature of man is Divine.

REST May 6

The pause that rests will heal most any condition if one is faithful to the Cause.

1 Becker page 25 Life in Motion, see also Bibliography and Notes

ZONE C May 7

Here we make friendships not bound by the persona of the culture.

ZONE C May 8

Groups sometimes form successfully to serve; institutions always fail from self-centeredness. The key to Zone C is service.

ZONE C May 9

The space that Zone C occupies depends on the nature of the service.

It can be a small room or the world; the Tide will show you the map in each event.

ZONE C May 10

It is ultimately the only Zone we have.

The other Zones have limits.
Zone C is our reverence for Life.
That Life is endless.

ZONE C May 11

Humility is the effect of being loved by the Tide and being changed.

Humility does not compare or contrast things. The duality ends and the world feels different.

ZONE C May 12

All of Osteopathy is Osteopathy.

Nothing else is.

REST May 13

Rest is a retreat into the interior world.

It is an opportunity to visit with the Health of the Truth that lives in us. One thing that can place us here is to be in the moment. This activity is not automatic but with the proper discipline it can place us in the arms of the Beloved. To be in the moment is to be outside of time in the movement of Creation, Love, and Eternity.

If we bring the senses into the present moment, very beautiful and interesting events occur. Let your eyes be aware of what is right here now. Let them see what is in your immediate environment and not wander into the past with imaginings and into the future with daydreams. Be here now, seeing what you see. Hold this awareness. Add the ears … listen only to the sound here now. Avoid listening to any inner dialogue about current or past events. Add touch … sense your body's position and activity while your eyes and ears are here also … add taste and smells.…

When sight, hearing and touch, are truly aligned with the moment, it will cause your attention to shift, without effort, into the Ocean and the movement of the Spirit of Life.

This is being present to the moment.… This is the incarnate movement of eternity and all of its agencies.

ZONE C May 14

The love for and from the Beloved gives birth to the memories of the Health.

We have two memories: one linear and subjective, one eternal and of the Health. Remembering the past is not real. It is self-centered. The truth can appear only here … now. You will find two lives in parallel; one needs a victim to exist, the other is in eternity and cannot be injured.

ZONE C May 15

Dr. Still wrote inside the cover of a student's book. "I love to love and be loved, do you?"

Mother Theresa of Calcutta wrote the purpose of life is "to love and be loved."[1]

What does this mean?

ZONE C May 16

Zone C begins to form when you develop an understanding of your limits in life.

We are very ignorant and self-serving … we need help. We must reach into the Sea, not our personal knowledge. For a physician to bow is right action. Service is done on the terms of the patient, not our analysis.

Listen.

1 Mother Theresa Nobel lecture given December 11, 1979

DECEPTION May 17

The application to Osteopathic School requires a statement of intent to be an Osteopath.

Most statements do not match the actions of the students who enter. I find this very odd. Has human nature lost its integrity? Is it now acceptable to lie on such an important statement? Or has it always been so?

DISCRIMINATION May 18

There is no going with the flow in Biodynamics.

One must discern the difference between lesion motion, the therapeutic force and the effects of transmutation.

How are these things different?

DISCRIMINATION May 19

There is healthy motion and unhealthy motion.

Our task is to discriminate one from the other. Lesion motions in the fluid body are not centered. Lesion motion does not cause the whole to shift in a new direction. Lesion motion lacks potency; its power is inertial. Lesion motions are repetitive and often have inhalation and exhalation patterns that are not mirror images. The fulcrum for the lesion motion is dead. If one directs the Tide gently the lesion does not alter itself. Lesions are not internally disengaging. If you are watching lesion motion there is no change in the autonomic nervous system until it begins to disengage or connect with Health and transmutate.

REST May 20

Rest brings about homeostasis, autonomic balance, emotional resolution, and neutrality.

It is necessary for a good healthy relationship with God, friends, family and oneself. Rest into a sacred place inside and feel the shelter.

DISCRIMINATION May 21

Every treatment is different.

Therapeutic forces have transmutative potency. There are infinite styles that the Tide can express. Our senses tell us that these forces come from outside the zones. We feel them arrive into the lesion field and then create effects that are in the part and in the whole as they move towards the Health. Therapeutic Forces are easily missed because they work so quickly. We tend to follow effects making for long treatments. When the therapeutic forces recede our job is finished, the effects may go on for days, weeks, or years.

WHEN IN DOUBT May 22

Go into deeper water.

WHEN YOU REACH YOUR LIMIT May 23

When you feel lost and at a dead end and you cannot find a sense of direction, ask for help from the "Other Pair of Hands."

The "Other Pair of Hands" is a reality that many elders spoke about when I interviewed them. Around 1987 I began to see the "Other Pair of Hands" when I was really lost and had used up my capacity to find a doorway to understand the treatment. I thought that I was having delusions but the clinical outcomes were dramatic. My sense of being taught during these events made me ask others about this.

Every one of the eight elders I spoke with, had definite experiences of the "Other Pair of Hands". The reports were so similar that I asked why no one had ever said anything. In one way or another they said fear of professional chastisement was the reason. This fear has plagued the growth of Osteopathy since its beginning.

I began to openly speak about the "Other Pair of Hands." Many were relieved to find out they were having a normal experience.

If you become quiet and wait, sensing the edge of the skin around the whole patient, the hands will be seen. You can learn great skill from them ... this skill is only momentary and is only for moments when you have reached you limit.

ABREACTION — May 24

This word has many uses.

The meaning I was given was spiritual in nature. The monastic use of the word means to move away from your reactivity to a stimulus. When one abreacts, one is actively passive. This leads eventually to the capacity to wait and not be so reactive to stimulation. Later it becomes patience and finally it grows into neutrality and an openness to the Will of the Tide.

Spiritual perception is not automatic; it is led by neutrality.

WAITING — May 25

Engagement of therapeutic forces requires waiting.

WAITING May 26

Fluid lesions have wave motion ... the unresolved.

You can be mesmerized by this motion and kept under a veil of doing. We are vulnerable to deception. Not all waves are therapeutic forces.

REST May 27

Rest builds a dependency on the Tide

WAITING May 28

Wait for the autonomics to balance, just wait ... then wait some more.

Try and see how the Tide is trying to create the balance. What is its method?

WAITING May 29

Wait in a healthy place ... there is a healthy place in the lesion.

There is a healthy place in you. There is a healthy place almost everywhere if we look for it.

WAITING May 30

Wait in the Meeting Place.

This is an indwelling room in your house designed for the purpose of contemplation and meeting the Master and leaving behind technique.

WAITING May 31

Concepts should not be active while one is waiting.

Patience is waiting outside of time. Do not work from motive. Observe your experience of patience. Is it empty?

Patience is waiting outside of time.

BE STILL AND KNOW June 1

These days as I teach in various places, I see many people attempting to 'be still and know'.

Their sincerity is very evident. Their understanding, however valid for them, is not what our teachers are pointing at when they said, "be still and know."

This phrase is part of a Hebrew chant, written by King David. The words 'be still and know' are not human in origin.

"Be still, and know that I am God;
I will be exalted among the nations,
I will be exalted in the earth!"[1]

God said, "Be still and know that I am God."[2] He was speaking to his beloved children. Stillness was created by God's breath

1 Psalm 46:10 New King James Version (NKJV) see Bibliography and Notes
2 ibid

as he spoke and his presence overshadowed everything. This overshadowing is unexpected and the voice is heard only by those who see God as the Beloved. When one is overshadowed, there is a profound sense of sanctification, purification, and of healing. One becomes a victim of love ... centered by the Divine. Love drowns out the stillness. Immobilized by God's will, one is still ... because God has stilled them in a profound meeting of longing. God makes the opening that allows himself to be known.

Be still is 'raphah' in Hebrew; it means to become or to let it drop ... drop what? Drop your claims on knowing, your will, your self-centering. God gives us the neutrality and transparency and being to hear his voice. This is considered by the great masters to be almost the final step in becoming. It is not a flux of our will to "be still and know" held by our intention, it is a miraculous opening into the Mystery of the Divine.

CO-EMERGENCE — June 2

All Laws pertaining to our existence co-emerge.

The Whole sprouts the whole ... unfolding does not end unless we become fixed. And so it is with children.

When you sense what appears to be one part, find the wholeness of its Health; follow this wholeness to the Whole.

REST — June 3

One is suspended in a more complete sense of life.

SYNCHRONIZATION June 4

Synchronize with something healthy.

This is where we begin. The patient enters; we see their Health. We ask how can I help you?

In the history we listen to the pauses and clarify the tiniest details. When we examine the patient we begin by sensing for something normal: the breathing of Primary Respiration, the Sea Around Us, the presence of the Tide, the Health.... Anything Beautiful!

This synchronizes us with Primary Respiration.

SYNCHRONIZATION June 5

It is easy just to follow motion and not see the stillness arise.

When we follow motion, without the stillness leading us, we are following lesions and not the therapeutic motion. Synchronization brings stillness into view. Make sure you look for this stillness to emerge into your awareness.

SYNCHRONIZATION June 6

When you find something to synchronize with, it must have meaning for you.

To just feel inhalation and exhalation, as a task, or a technique, is not true involvement with the Health. Look for something that strikes your heart ... that somehow awakens you to beauty. This is not a skill; it is a livingness that is inside you.

You will find inner peace from that beauty.

SYNCHRONIZATION June 7

Sometimes we are already synchronized and we do not know it because we are not sensing the Health in us, but rather looking at our limits.

Look inside behind the veil of your mental aberrations ... are you already synchronized? Many students synchronize because they think they are not perfect and, miss the point. This will create fatigue and some tensions at bedtime. Perhaps synchronization is already active in your heart. Assuming you are not perfect is overdoing what is not true.

SYNCHRONIZATION June 8

I am walking around, considering how to fix a sprinkler.

Then a liquid light comes into me from what appears to be outside. I stop. I am transmutated, synchronized by a spontaneous healing from the hand of the Master. I fix the sprinkler without any to-do. The Health is foremost in my perception.

Gratitude is innocent, not full of emotion, neutral.

SYNCHRONIZATION June 9

First do no harm, by forcing your attention on the patient.

Respect the need for help and assume it comes for everyone.

REST June 10

The breathing contains several motions.

During the inhalation phase, the beginning is just before the diaphragm begins to move. It is a soft sweet tensionless motion.... Find this and stay with it. Let the breathing continue but place your attention here. Doing this will bring changes and rest.

SYNCHRONIZATION June 11

First do no harm.

Do not synchronize with the person or their thoracic respiration. As nice as this seems it is a means of creating dependency and weak boundaries. You could imprint, lose yourself and not know it.

SYNCHRONIZATION June 12

Synchronization occurs around a Midline that is independent of any persona or personal goals.

TEETH June 13

The growth and development of teeth involves incredible motion, timing, spatial orientation, and fluid body activity.

Dentition is not a mechanically driven event. If you can find pictures of all the stages of dentition, beginning with the buds that are embryonic, you will see a precision of activity that Osteopathy is built upon. Carefully studied, you will see that upper and lower teeth have a midline that they share. Each tooth and its partner are on one axis. Knowing this helps in treatment of displaced teeth, delayed progress of growth and in the evaluation of function.

Find the local midline, sense both the teeth and the potency of their shared midline and see what you think.

THE MANDIBLE June 14

As students, generally we are trained that the mandible is one bone. Magoun, on page 201 in Osteopathy in the Cranial Field 3rd edition, reveals a mechanistic model that states the mandible is not part of the face, but is mechanically moved by the temporals and the occiput, not the sphenoid. He also considers it one bone, not two. This view has many flaws and a review of the developmental fluid fields of the mandibular arch will give a different picture.

The mandible, like the frontal bone, is two bones; they move as paired bones in the adult as well as the child. These two bones should share a single fulcrum and a single motion towards lamina terminalis during the involuntary inhalation phase. Normal motion is a receding towards lamina terminalis during inhalation with a widening across the transverse axis. It gets shorter and fatter, so to speak. However, the two sides often have very different patterns.

The mandible has three dimensional internal motion that is whole. When lesioned it can take on very distorted unilateral intra-osseous motion. If one synchronizes with the motion present during the inhalation phase therapeutics will occur and demonstrate what we propose as the normal physiological motions.

THERAPEUTICS June 15

Synchronization with the motion in the lesion during the inhalation period triggers a therapeutic process that begins with 2 1/2 cycles per minute and can end at a much deeper endpoint. The inhalation phase is one of internal disengagement. Synchronization with motion present creates more disengagement. The Tide is directing its potency and at the same time bringing augmentation, transmutation, synchronization and disengagement together as one event ... very powerful principles at work. This is the activity of the inhalation phase and why we use it.

NATURAL PERCEPTION June 16

We are endowed with senses ... perceptual doorways.

Children grow by the impressions received. Synapses form at an enormous rate—millions per minute in the first years of life. We lose 60% of these connections from disuse. As we move away from our natural state our senses loose their broadness.

We enter school, and over many years, we lose natural instinct and passive sensation. This intensifies during higher education and limits our capacity to interface with natural laws and understand Osteopathy. We need to teach children to continue to develop their natural mind as they begin to make academic efforts.

Teaching rational palpation is unnatural because the senses have been reversed and supervised by mental concepts. Our task, as teachers of Osteopathy, is to renew the broadness of perception so that interested students can begin to return to a more healthy and natural state of engaging patients.

Spend time not directing your senses towards the obvious. Wait and let your attention come back to its natural fulcrum—that of neutrality.

REST June 17

Resting lengthens your life ....

Rest refreshes your autonomics ... just watch your pulse and respirations express relief as you rest. Resting is a lost art; it is a principle of Osteopathy and life.

PALPATION AND SENSING June 18

Palpation is an attempt to be efferent and touch things to see if they match a model that is learned.

Sensing is afferent and involves being alert to what is being sensed by the mind. The mental shift from palpation to sensing contradicts the generally accepted doctor image and authoritarian mindset that many hide behind out of fear that their ignorance may be displayed.

Palpation is Newtonian and fits into the ideas of mechanics that structuralists prefer. Sensing is a fearless receptivity of something new. Just as Sutherland and his study group all had to make this shift, so do most Osteopath's coming out of training today. Our bodies, and our patients' bodies also, feel the difference in our touch; when we are sensing it experienced as more relaxing and healthy.[1]

Sit and let your senses come to center ... notice how you feel and behave.

1 See Notes and Bibliography

SUTHERLAND June 19

Sutherland went well beyond the mechanical model and palpation.

He set aside gears and levers and found a direct communication with Primary Respiration. In his study group and with his students, this is what he taught. This communication is the basis of our work.

Osteopathic training institutions are afraid of nature; we invent allopathic models for what reason? We are weak. We are afraid we will be condemned. To be an Osteopath is to choose a different model for healing, one that works even better than the allopathic model in a general practice.

Cranial motion is life - not physics.... Sutherland set the mechanical aside once he saw the intelligence of the fluids

EYES OPEN June 20

In my study group with Dr. Becker he taught us to sense.

He taught us to wait, to listen, to be neutral and to be still and hear "the still small voice of God".[1] In an effort to be more passive, we closed our eyes during treatments. This went on for several years. One day Dr. Becker said "now do it with your eyes open". This was really hard, but after a few years, the veil lifted; we could see the Tide.

The invisible was visible in both worlds....

RATES AND DISCERNMENT June 21

Primary Respiration is subtle and at best difficult to observe and interpret.

Mental activity in oneself or the patient makes for a tedious and vague understanding of the intention of the Tide in the

1 1 Kings 19:12 King James Version (KJV)

moment. This mental activity makes the waters opaque and forces one to motion test and use force. At quieter mental proportions and slower rates the water becomes more and more transparent and more detail becomes evident.

An excited mind or faster rates, more than 3 cycles per minute, will make clarity impossible, making one dependent on palpation and direct action. At slower rates the mind is afferent and listening with the hands.

COMPRESSION OF THE RECIPROCAL TENSION POTENCY

June 22

The reciprocal tension potency (R.T.P.) is the fluid in the fluid.

Sutherland described it as an electromagnetic force. There were fluctuations of this potency. He called these the longitudinal and lateral fluctuations. He saw these fluctuations as direct and alternating currents, respectively. He also described the steady state of fluctuation in the whole as breathing.

If you compress the R.T.P. the result is varied. It could inhibit the therapeutic forces and prolong the treatment. It could make the patient feel as if you were pushing on them, as if your hands were too forceful. It could increase the rate of Primary Respiration. It could inhibit the neutral in the whole from occurring easily. It could produce an autonomic storm with emotional liabilities. It usually takes a teacher to notice that you are compressing the R.T.P. Seeing it for yourself, without help, is rare, because it is not easy to identity. When it happens in a course, the label of hypersensitive is placed on the student being treated when in fact the operator is invasive. Often it comes from going too deep too fast. Ask a friend or Biodynamic teacher to check you out for this habit; it will save you travail later.

The treatment for a compression of the RTP is simple if one avoids measures, like CV4, that control the RTP. Go to the Health, the Liquid Light, and the sensation of love passing through it and wait without trying to help.

When we think orthopedics, we are not thinking Osteopathy.[1]

In 1986 a middle-aged woman came to see me with a chief complaint of a right-sided Bell's Palsy. It had begun 8 weeks before. Besides her family doctor, she had seen a neurologist and unsuccessfully taken a steroid dose-pack.

I explained to her that I was going use my hands to check her system and take more history at the next visit. I did this because she had seen two good physicians and also because the Tide would provide the diagnostics ... if I stayed away from assumptions.

I began by listening to the Health and letting the Tide make the decisions. Slowly, the patient went to a neutral. Her fluid body was balanced and peaceful. I waited for the diagnostics from the Tide. The therapeutic forces began working near her right ovary. From a fulcrum in that area there was a clear lesion field on the whole left trunk that was a flaccid fluid field with distinct boundaries. The Tide worked there and then I could feel a reflexive release of the eyes and sub-occipital muscles.

I questioned her about her ovaries. She said that she had polycystic ovarian disease. Further questioning revealed severe psychological trauma when her ovulatory cycles began at age 12.

As usual, I called her in three days. She was asymptomatic. She did not need further treatment.

Lesions are in the whole, not the part. The facial nerve was not addressed nor did it need to be.
Can you imagine the whole lesioning and not having cause where the orthopedic model suggests?

1 Sutherland page 211 second edition Contributions of Thought

REST — June 24

Rest can be accessed through listening to the pauses in the conversation with the patient.

CASES THAT INFORM — June 25

In 1978 a sixty-seven year old surgeon came to see me with Bell's Palsy.

He has been disabled for 6 months. He had seen many doctors and taken steroids. He was no better and said he wanted "cranial work." I told him I was going to listen to his system, treat him and then hope that would unveil the cause. Once in neutral the Tide went straight to his first rib on the right and his cervico-thoracic junction. It was there a long time … it stalled. I manually put the rib and vertebra in neutral using the direction of ease ... the Tide continued to hammer away at this one place. I waited for ten minutes. The patient took a deep breath and concurrently went to a complete neutral in the whole.

He called the next day and was asymptomatic. He never had any further problems.

CASES THAT INFORM — June 26

In 1988 an 84-year-old woman came to see me with Bell's palsy.

She had been symptomatic for seventeen years with classical symptoms. I was saying to myself that I could not help her. I treated her with the same principles I have in other cases—first neutral, then wait for the Tide to demonstrate its diagnostics. She went to neutral easily but stayed for a long time ... a long time. Then nothing else. I was sure she was not going to be helped. I called her in three days. She was 30% better. I was very surprised but remained outwardly calm. Two more treatments over several months created no additional changes. She was much happier because now she could close her eye which had not closed for seventeen years. Her corneal dryness had ended and she could smile a lot better.

Live and learn … there is a wholeness.

CASES THAT INFORM — June 27

In 1988 a 55 year old woman with a stiff back, hip pain and a loss of vitality came to see me.

This patient has accessed many physicians for help, so I told her I was going to leave out the history and ask her questions as the Tide illuminated certain facts.

I began by listening to the whole and she went to a neutral easily. Then I placed my hands under her lumbar spine and listened. The Tide outlined a lesion field and then went through the fulcrum to another lesion field without treating. The next lesion field demonstrated poor muscle tone in the legs and a fulcrum in her throat and thyroid. I asked if she had ever had a thyroid problem. "Yes," she answered, she had been on thyroid medication for 10 years. Then the Tide went into her head and it lit up. I asked her if she had ever seen a light and she told me about two near drownings as a youth that were accompanied by a sense of peaceful transcendence and light. That ended the visit. I was not sure if she had really treated.

When she returned in a week she was more vital, her muscle tone was much better and her back stiffness had eased … only her hips remained painful. The ignition in her head was still very bright so I did not treat her. The same was true on the next visit.

What I believed happened in these first few visits was that the event of seeing the light in her near drownings had stayed with her all these years. It had waited until she was free to treat her foundational lesion— one that I never saw. She, however, in addition to decreased pain reported awareness of certain psychological tendencies that changed in all this.

CONCLUSIONS REACHED BY DEDUCTION ARE LIMITED

June 28

We must learn to "Think Osteopathy." [1]*How do we get to the Teacher?*

Still and Sutherland claimed to be led ... to follow a Superior Intelligence.
This Superior Intelligence is indwelling, that is our professional premise.
How does one meet the Tide and its intelligence?

BONES

June 29

To understand bones, one must look beyond the anatomical position.

Learn how each bone is made, how it is shaped and the origin of its position. Learn its history and how it maintains it's internal wholeness and integrity. Know what a bone is guided by.

What holds the lesion inside the bone?

CAUSE

June 30

Can we find the Intelligence and that creates, compensates and heals?

It is not outside itself but inside the bone?

1 Sutherland page 211 second edition Contributions of Thought

REST July 1

The first part of the inhalation phase of Thoracic Respiration is without tension.

At the immediate beginning of thoracic inhalation there is no resistance. In the next part there is a crescendo of tension. Notice the ease at the beginning and keep your mind on it ... you will REST and witness many deep truths.

SELF July 2

The Self that precedes the immune system has no location.

It gives rise to the self/non-self interface. The Self draws and molds the body, the physiology and brain into form. It awakens the fluid we call protoplasm. This Self is the Health or the True Self and has no anatomical place where one could find it; rather it is in the Whole. When we sense its presence we feel incredible love and permanence.

SANCTUARY July 3

Your treatment room will become a silent mirror.

Having a reflective environment in which to work requires personal attention to the quality and atmosphere of the treatment room. My treatment room is a sacred space where I give myself 100 percent to God and this work. I clean it and care for it; the room is like a church for me. It helps me remember my responsibility and aim. When I am off center I go there and it quiets me. Attend to your treatment space and over time your room will build character and will heal you.

Each night as you close the door you will feel the Health.

REBALANCING July 4

Rebalancing should be the first principle taught in all courses.

Every year there are students who are injured during basic courses in which rebalancing is not taught. I know because I treat many of these people. Please promote safety. Rebalancing is an act of humility.

QUESTION July 5

Do you think there is a gene for wholeness?

STOP July 6

Stop self-intervention; it will not heal anything.

Trying to analyze yourself is a vicious circle of lesioning. The Tide can lead you to the place of transmutation. Your own plan is coming from your ego and as such will keep you in repetition.

FATIGUE July 7

At the end of the day, light a candle in your office.

Return after awhile and extinguish it. This clears the heart

REST July 8

The final resting place is the Health.

Death is not the end. The more one prepares for death the less meaning it has as something unpleasant. Rest and ponder your death without thinking. Just enter the question.

VARIABILITY July 9

Variability should be written as one of the laws of healing.

Techniques usually assume that the patient is normal or the lesion is stupid. Because we use our hands to engage therapeutics we need to think about the presence of variability in patients and lesions. I do not use techniques for several reasons—this being one of them.

Variability is rarely taken into the foreground of our thinking but variability is what we are witnessing in every case. If we do not know how to interact with variability then we will get results that are contradictory. For example: if you want to do a CV4 you apply the technique in a fashion you prefer. Then you may or may not see the results.

If you don't see results, answer these questions: Did you adjust your mental intentions to meet the fact that the supraocciput is rarely symmetrical? What if one O-M is lesioned and the other is free? Every patient will be a variation, not a norm and so we must meet the variation, and adjust our technique so as not to override the variation. Our technique is often asymmetrical ... as it should be.

I remember in 1974 I was trying to do a frontal lift on a patient. As I disengaged the sutures with internal rotation in preparation for the lift, the left side was so lesioned it would not disengage ... so I lifted what would lift and ended up with a slanted disengagement. As I waited, the Tide centered the therapeutic force to the slanted position rather than centering the bone. Then I understood who really knew technique! Do not plow through variations, bring variations into the technique and adjust your feeling fingers and your intentions accordingly. The Tide will demonstrate the skill to accommodate the variations.

VARIABILITY — July 10

The pattern of inertia in a lesion field is variable. No two strains have the same geometry. One vertical strain is not like any other vertical strain. We must feel the variability in order not to disturb the fluids or worse, the brainstem. Variation is part and parcel of the lesion; it gives us a sense of direction that could be missed with a technique that uses force.

VARIABILITY — July 11

Anatomy is never like what is in the books ...

There is a dynamic of life and very little adynamic anatomy. Finding a fascial plane in a healthy person in a relaxed state is a challenge, why?

VARIABILITY — July 12

The Tide never treats the same way twice. The principles of treatment change from minute to minute. I guarantee that if you are not alert, you will cause the tempo of the therapeutics to lesion. Unfortunately, if you follow the Tide in the direction you anticipate from past experience; the rate will change and the outcome will be disappointing.

VARIABILITY July 13

Your awareness is not consistent; if you try and make it that way you will become a robot. Perception automatically shifts; it never repeats itself. We foolishly think it does.

TRANSMUTATION July 14

During the inhalation period of Primary Respiration the sphenoid becomes transparent and one sees liquid light. We cannot see these things unless we are centered by the Tide and are aware of It as our Cause.

REST July 15

Do something different ...

Behave in a new manner
Rest from your self.
Turn left when you feel to turn right
... just once
...what happens?

WISE WORDS July 16

"When all the fulcrums are synchronized there will be peace and harmony"[1]

Dr. Sutherland is very clear about a picture of normal. Have you felt this? It is a picture of wholeness.

1 Sutherland See Bibliography and Notes

WISE WORDS July 17

Our skill is proportionate to our understanding of Normal[1]

Dr. Still points us towards the Health. How do you picture normal? Your sense of normal may limit the transmutative process. Really feel into the question...what does it feel like to be normal?

THE POINT July 18

"Do you see the point?"[2]

I believe that Sutherland knew that the manifested activity of a certain quality of Health had a fulcrum from which that function unfolded. To find the fulcrum and witness its meaning removed the dross from the activity and allowed one to see more of the Reality.

Ruby talked a lot about Sutherland or 'Will,' as she called him. In this study group, Ruby told me, between 1935-1954, Will would teach a single topic and after a least a year of daily applications when the group had mastered it and were in the wholeness of the principle ... he would say, "Do you see the point?" Ruby reported this experience in her first class with Will. It was 1935, she was in her forties, and she had traveled a long way by rail to get to the course. For seven days they worked to have complete a picture of the CV4. This was all that was taught during the whole week. Then she went home and used the principle for a year. When she returned to the group, at the endpoint of a practical, Will said, "Do you see the point?"

From my conversations with Ruby I believe he meant, "Did you find the fulcrum which generated the entire wholeness of a particular process?" Once the fulcrum was found a new landscape appeared. This is how he moved forwards.

---

1 Still Page

2 Sutherland, Day See Bibliography and Notes

Once you have a skill, the skill must die so you can grow. Finding the point does this. As it does, your impressions change and you move forward, with precision, into deeper water. You are alone in undiscovered country. This method is powerful and difficult. You may come to that think you do not know anything. In a sense you do not and in a sense you can choose to know or not, and not knowing opens a doorway to an Ocean

THE POINT — July 19

Everything you perceive is from one point;

All motion is from one point. You can witness this, but to get to that place you must travel past many interior landscapes.

You must pass through many losses.

Your expert must die over and over and over, then the Master will open your heart for you to see, through His eyes. He will show you what is occurring in the whole of Life.

Like Dante you travel, not alone, but with help always near.

TEMPO — July 20

The natural and divine worlds are a single event expressing life in a profoundly synchronized manner according to a timetable that remains hidden in mystery.

When we enter the landscape of a single moment we must try and remember that we are not God, the healer. We are not the origin of the insight necessary for the conclusive result that we anticipate in our ignorance. We enter the moment as part of life, unaware of our particular consciousness until it is raised up by, and with, the Whole. The Whole brings every element of being, from star to darkness, into a relationship of change.

Our job is not to heal but to observe the movement that carries our awareness into transmutation.

TEMPO

July 21

Life is rhythmic. It has a tempo.

Small simple motions will yield great results if they are in tempo with the intention of the Tide. Tempo is the gait of manifestation, it saunters. It does not rush to overcome. It seeks balance, not victory... balancing the whole into the Whole ... it uses power that in seconds does the impossible. It transmutates faster than your mind can see. Tiny motions, tiny little movements that are in tempo with the Intention of Primary Respiration, will yield results that seem miraculous. Sutherland mentioned 1/1000 of an inch as enough movement to be an effective treatment.

Watch for these tiny movements and follow.

REST

July 22

Meet with others of the same disposition ... it will replenish your soul. Meet and linger.

LIMITS

July 23

Dr. Rollin. Becker, in his moments of directness, reminded us to be less self-directed. He said to keep it simple. If someone needs something simple then give it to her instead of going into deep esoteric complexities. Sometimes, we believe that going deep is a skill that will yield more results. Sometimes, we think we are deep when in fact we are more superficial because a false fulcrum has been created.

Meet the Tide where it is.

LIMITS July 24

We focus on depth when a simple act would do.

We focus on having the answer for another's travail when a simple question could bring the Tide's full power. We avoid simplicity by setting ourselves outside the moment. We lock in like a guided missile because we think there is a dividing wall. The question is, who is separate and why? We separate because we want the power of being the healer.... This contradicts Osteopathy.

LIMITS July 25

Osteopathy is a visionary act.

To prematurely focus on something in the patient creates subliminal chaos; then it appears to the ego that the patient will not get well for some psychological reason but in essence we have upset the time clock and altered the tempo of the Tide's intention in this world.

HUMILITY July 26

Humility begins when we serve a tempo that is not our own.

It is hard trying to serve another's will that is in motion, but that is the task. Serve another's tempo and you will find gold in your inner world. Try this at home in little things and you will become amazed at what you understand. Someone suggests a place to eat supper. Go where they wish without any resistance or comment. Be neutral. Follow a little and a door will swing open.

NOTATION July 27

A true neutral makes the ego think, 'why am I so weak?'

The ego can be afraid of the quality of the docility as the muscles refuse to work for it. The muscles go limp, like water, the body seems to be empty of tension. The ego thinks, 'something is wrong with me.'

There is a Healthy surprise awaiting you.

CRUCIATE SUTURE July 28

At the center of the cruciate suture is a fulcrum, a point that appears before the form. From the center point of the cruciate suture one can appreciate a vertical line—a line of many points. There are force vectors from every point that create the anatomical relationships in the Fluid Body.

The four bones are created around the fulcrum. The shapes of the bones are there in the fluid before the bone precipitates. Look at the beauty. Forget the words and the anatomy. Look at it and feel it as if it was transparent to a higher function. Growth occurs but the point never moves!

Here is a place of exact fact.
Exact facts, seen correctly, empty the mind of the fog of structure.

REST July 29

"You can always count on anatomy to take you straight through to Grace." [1]

But you must drop the anatomy.

---

1 Jennifer Weiss, D.O.

ESSENTIALS

July 30

Dr. Wales repeated, over and over, to her students: "We are a living organism. We need air, water, food and shelter."[1]

I would often just let the words pass, not attending to them. She said it at so many meetings that I stopped listening. The metaphor was so deep that I missed the content.

We need air, water, food and shelter. This is an essential principle, important for every patient.

We need air, water, food and shelter. Let the words sink to the bottom of the well inside your heart. Let the words reach to their origin.

THE CLAVICLE

July 31

Dr. Fulford said once that he thought the clavicle was a cranial bone.

He made me think, "Is it?" Its location and shape, seem to be related to the upper extremity, not the cranium, but from where does the tissue originate?

What does embryology show us?

The clavicle is the first bone to begin ossification. The bone, which forms in membrane, has an outer layer, an inner layer, and a fluid field. These layers can lesion separately.

Ossification, with growth centers that form around a midline axis, begins from the center and spreads to the ends of the bone. Final stages begin around the age of fifteen, starting from the ends and moving towards the center. The periosteum is innervated by the 11th cranial nerve; this gives the key to its origin.

The bone straight, then curves to match the curvature of the innominate crest in the pelvis. As it curves its midline axis

1 See Bibliography and Notes

does not shift. As the clavicle grows, the sternocleidomastoid and the trapezius separate, having been one muscle before the bone lengthened and curved.

The clavicle is a fulcrum for the movement and development of the temporal bones, the thorax, and the shoulder. It interacts with the activities of all these structures. It dances with the involuntary movement of the shoulder, Thoracic Respiration and Primary Respiration.

The clavicle is commonly stressed at birth. If a child cries when picked up, check for a fracture.

If one feels the midline for the growth and development of the clavicle, and disregards knowledge of anatomy, then the fluid will correct dysfunction, giving rise to remolding and repositioning. It is quite something to watch.

These words are not designed to prove anything. The words express the awe and love I see in this beautiful living form — form that minute to minute wants to be perfectly balanced.

You can easily feel these things, if you leave the anatomy behind and feel the yearning of the form to be perfect and rest in its original pattern.

BALANCED FLUID TENSION August 1

A frozen shoulder, tissue scaring from chemotherapy, radiation, or surgery all have "withering fields".[1] When we examine these cases, the tissue is hard and barren of physiology. There is no life force or involuntary motion. Post mastectomy upper extremity dysfunction responds well to treatment using fluid dynamics. Balanced fluid tension will accomplish much more than direct action, and faster in all these cases.

Here is an approach: define the boundary of the lesion field. It can be extensive. At the edge of the lesion field, or sometimes in it, you will find fluid motion that is synchronized with the breathing of the Tide. During the inhalation phase the fluid will make a shape that is distorted or off midline. During exhalation instead of a return, the lesion field makes another distorted shape. Treatment occurs when the operator synchronizes with the tempo and shape change of the inhalation motion present in the fluid. Self-correcting forces take over and bring the part back to the whole.

THE HIDDEN August 2

When engaging a part, one must be thinking and prepared for the therapeutic process to move to an unexpected location, potentially distant from where one is working. For example, as I was treating a frozen shoulder using the fluid motion present at the interface between the inertia and momentum, there was a change. I was all ready to go to the clavicle when the Tide moved the potency of the therapeutic process to the sacrum. I watched and waited. Then the Tide went back to the area on the anterior surface of the scapula. The patient's frozen shoulder resolved. I still was thinking "clavicle!"

Somehow the Tide sees us much differently than we do … the sequence of prioritization is a mystery

How can one enter the Teaching of the Tide?

---

1 Still page 39 Philosophy of Osteopathy See Bibliography and Notes

CONVERSION

August 3

Once the senses are converted by the Teacher, the Teacher becomes more direct and the observer enters a living wholeness. This requires an understanding of third level stillness and a love for the Health as a living friend. The Teacher is not of this world.

LESSONS

August 4

A 56 year old woman comes to see me with a chief complaint of intractable sciatica. She had been a patient of my father 40 years earlier. She has had back surgery and many consults with biomechanical specialists. She is an inspiration as a person of simplicity and kindness.

I found a lesion in the sacral region that felt intra-osseous. I engaged it with motion present. Things went well. I could see the sequence and it made sense.
She returned in a week. "How are you?" I asked. "My back is no better," she said. I was disappointed. I was so sure I had done a good job. Then, she took off her socks and showed me 4 large ulcerations on her ankles. "Look," she said, "my ulcers are filling in." I saw craters filling with granulation tissue. I paused. I had not seen the ulcers on the first visit. "I have had these for ten years and I go every week for debridement and dressing. They have never filled before. My doctor said it was impossible. I had no surgical debridement this time." She was smiling and happy. I was dumbfounded.

I then, with great self-doubt, focused on her back. I went to the pelvis and waited. The fluid went to work, as it did she said, "it feels like during labor when my back was hurt." I was holding myself still out of fear that I might distort the treatment.

After she left, I sat a long time in my chair meeting my ignorance and crying softly. I felt a betrayal of a part of myself I did not know well.

I knew that she has been treated by the Tide and that I had missed the whole thing in my arrogance. I was coming to a choice about awareness. It was 1979. Her ulcers healed very well as did her sciatica.

Osteopathy has saved my soul from self-destruction.

REST

August 5

Rest can occur verbally.

Just wait before you engage an event by speaking.

LESSONS

August 6

In 1982 a 40 year old patient with a history of leukemia, bilateral acoustic neuromas, subdural hematomas, deep vein thrombosis and severe headaches came to see me. She had a hematocrit of three and was taking multiple medications. I was listening to all these things as I sat with her. They were happening to her all at once. She wanted Osteopathy to help her wholeness gather momentum. I agreed to try.

"Let's see what happens," I said. She lay down. I intentionally felt no lesions; I listened to the Health and waited in the quiet. The Tide did something in another room in the House Under the Sea.[1] She received a lot of help from the Tide. Over the next several years, she became well. She came every three months

I have no idea what transpired in her treatments, but I was coming to a place of neutrality in my perception. Neutrality is a doorway to the Teacher. It requires a big change. One must love the Tide unconditionally.

1 See Bibliography and Notes

A STORY

August 7

A poor woman, framed and bent with time, walking home peacefully after dark, to a single candled-room.

One candle, a holy light,
night,
and silence.

Her worn clothing dances in the light as she sits alone eating, her heart peaceful in the sanctuary of simplicity.

Years of living and hardship, children now grown, her husband dead from despair. She sits.

One candle light,
the night,
the stillness.

Overhead in the night-sky an angel watches.

"It is I sitting there, finally without pain", the angel says to himself, as he feels the holy light from her window, like a beacon into the darkened sky. "I," he says, "it is I, finally without despair."

Dawn rises. The candle ends with a gentle sweep of her breath.

Stillness,
Daylight,
time passing.

The door opens almost by itself. She rises, walks through it into the street, returning again to work.

Nothing shifts inside her as she walks, bent forwards.

The rising sun breathes into her worn clothes and the fire touches Itself.

THE EGO August 8

The word has many definitions. The one used here is that the ego is a self—a destructive false self that is hidden in the subconscious. It controls us without our awareness of it.

All of my mentors felt strongly that we all must seek out our ego in order to have real freedom, the freedom to choose our responses to circumstances, not be a slave to synapses. Pride, envy, resentment are certainly characteristics of the ego but my search has been for more subtle activities that precede our fall into the ego's domain.

Once you have felt a deep neutral in yourself, you will have more certainty about when your ego is in control and when you are being moved towards the Health. Being neutral is the freedom to move in the direction of the Health, with ease. And the tone of that dynamic ease is not present when self interest is the fulcrum.

THE EGO August 9

In 2001 I took a ten-day retreat to study as many manuscripts as possible that considered the ego. I was searching for ways to tell when the ego was around that were subtle and more easily overlooked until it was too late to be neutral. Here are some points I gleaned from the retreat.

The ego will not rest—it keeps going and going. It is on barrier no matter how justifiable the motive appears, if you feel barrier in your self, even at your center, it is the ego.

It fears greatly humiliation.

It fabricates.

It is self-centered like the early belief that the earth was the center of the solar system.

It creates linear time.

It defines spaces through ownership ... my house, my car, my teaching, my child, et cetera

The ego lacks refined sensory skills. It will not cross into the unknown without force, thusly distorting the new landscape.

Suffering is to be avoided and denied for pleasure.

It must be the savior.

It makes one clever.

It refuses the third principle as leadership.

It must always gain ground.

It thinks it can find God.

It thinks it is the Whole.

It uses the senses to prove others are wrong.

It sorts memories into good and bad.

It is unaware of tempo from others. It cannot love.

It forgets even the greatest moments of Divine Love.

The sensation of neutral and the sensation of a prowler in the house are accurate enough to keep you alert and free, if you wish. The ego actually makes a disturbance you can appreciate that is not a thought or an emotion...

SEAMS — August 10

Seams are different than segments in that they are not related to the notochord.

They are the folding of the whole, geometrically related to the central midline. They are one alleyway ... not many separate seams.

SEAMS August 11

The seam that becomes the boundary between the frontal and temporal lobes is one of the lines that patterns the anterior dural fluid field.

It arises from pre-sphenoid protoplasm. The space opens and a shape appears.

REST August 12

Falling in Love with the Living God in all things is a source of great relief when we sit.

THE MOTION PRESENT August 13

The involuntary motion in tissue is an effect of Primary Respiration.

We call it 'motion present' to differentiate it from 'motion permitted,' which is an effect of the introduction of force by a clinician.

The pattern and influence of the motion upon its immediate environment is a manifestation of the degree of health it can express. A normal pattern is related to the central midline and is synchronized with the breathing of Primary Respiration. Normal tissue motion transmutates, that is, it changes to a fluid state at the end of inhalation. Normal tissue motion is also synchronized with the fluid transmutation and the transmutation of the fluid in the fluid.

The exchange of momentum between biological compartments is called augmentation. As these compartments approach neutral, they come to a balance point and homogenize into a neutral state that goes still. They re-awaken as a single unit of life with a slower rate or no rate at all. With time the tissue, fluid and potency can return to a single substance that is transparent and reflects the Health more completely.

DOORWAYS

August 14

The sutures of the cranium move.

They are not gears that transfer motion from the base, the vault, the face and the sacrum. The sutures are one suture, a matrix of interconnected design that allows motion to occur. The sutures open, then the bones breathe into the space created. The shape change occurs everywhere, in brain, fluid and connective tissue.

Space opens, then function moves in ... this is embryology ... in an embryo and in an adult.

The idea of an R.T.M. moving the bones is outdated. Sutherland abandoned it in 1953. It was reductionistic and linear. Remember that in children the sutures are not serrated, they are smooth along all edges, so the idea of the gearing mechanism is not a theoretical possibility in children.

DROPS

August 15

Every drop knows the Tide[1]

A drop ... one drop. How big is a drop?
Rain drops, tear drops spherical drops. Smallness. Drops of dew. Drops of oil.
A drop ... inside is a living embryo ... sheltered.
A small being floating in one drop of sea water, sheltered in a sphere.

STOP THE PIA

August 16

One day, in a study group, Ruby Day began talking about the motion of the brain, the reciprocal tension membrane and the bones. She went to the sacrum of my fellow student. She said, "Watch the mechanism." I had my hands on the head. All of a sudden the brain halted its motion, as did the bones, but the

1 See Bibliography and Notes

fluid kept fluctuating. She was excited and said, "there."

I was not sure what she was pointing out. I felt mentally dazed by her words. I waited. She could see my dullness.

"Will showed me that!" she exclaimed. She then explained. "Will showed us how to stop the CNS motion by holding the filum terminale at the sacral attachment.

Sutherland had figured out how to test his theory and it proved wrong. He was delighted by what he learned. The theory was that the reciprocal tension membrane was moved by the brain and the RTM moved the fluids. Ruby went on, "I inhibit the pia, then the brain and bones stop moving, but the fluids keep fluctuating ... that means that the fluid is not moved by the RTM." She was ecstatic.

His theory was found to be in error. She and Will were joyful.

"Why be happy about failure?" I thought. "Besides I never really paid any attention to the RTM and the fluid...what's the big deal?"

Will and his friends were seekers of truth—not theories. As they often said, "we want to communicate with the real thing, not laws framed by human hands." When the Tide brought them closer to understanding the mechanism that was all they wanted— intimacy. Their ideas could die but to be closer to the Mystery; that was exciting. They had no investment other than seeing more deeply into creation.

I was thirty-six. The lesson was over my head. I went home and studied the theory of the RTM and the fluid; then I was silent and sad ... sad for the time I had wasted wanting the right answer and missing the journey into beauty.

Ruby was with Will a long time. She loved his teaching and his unquenchable thirst for real water.

HOUSE CALLS

August 17

In 1971 a house call was five dollars. It was the same wherever the call took me, five miles or thirty miles. The time alone in my truck driving through the back roads of rural Maine, in the forest and along clear streams, was not a burden. Often, I stopped and ate my lunch, had a coffee and found time for my spirit.

The patients were usually unable to leave their houses and yet needed regular visits for chronic illnesses. With rare exception, I was welcomed with warmth and gratitude.

I wanted to learn from them about their lives and the past that they had journeyed. Rural America is full of self-sufficient individuals with skills that were, even then, almost lost.

I learned a lot about homesteading, fishing, tool use, cooking with wood, and every aspect of nature. It was a joyful task to ride into another world and help people who had no cars and needed care.

I never felt burdened and the five dollars was a plus.

No one went without care or medications and there were no government programs. The town pharmacist and the drug companies donated what medications were needed. Neighbors were charitable in heart and time. There were no excesses or abuse except for a few alcoholics who did not know any better.

Then came Medicare. The federal government regulations came with a destruction of a culture. We were regulated to the point where a nurse from a corporate business was required to see the patient first, before we could go out on a call. It was a big business that had gotten into our simple system. The charge for the nurse was 45 dollars; the government then paid us 9 dollars for our house call services. The new wave of corporate government was invading the idea of love your neighbor, something the rural people in their pride did so well.

A simple human interchange died as the whole mechanized

system destroyed the soul of a little outpost of humanitarian culture. The benefit to the people was nothing. The quality of health care declined because the heart felt connection within the community was killed in the name of progressive health care.

The next generation did not make house calls.

The urban values came into remote areas like a cancer; it killed the grace, instinct and service innate to the people and their community life.

MIGNE — August 18

Let that by which you are wounded become your cure.[1]

When it cures you it is because you have learned to love the cause.

REST — August 19

We can lean on the knowledge that the Health has Wisdom.

It can give you love and rest. This is why different levels of stillness are vital. Discernment is not the most refined mental tool ...Wisdom is.

TRANSVERSE MOTION — August 20

You can study your mental orientation by observing lateral motion in the therapeutics.

Lateral motion occurs along a transverse plane relative to the midline. It is not a lateral fluctuation. Being alert to transverse motions helps to expose any tendency one has to 'look at the

1 Jacques Paul Migne

center or midline of the patient and lock up the fluid body.

The tendency to look down the midline is a foundational skill in biomechanics, but with the Fluid Body it is disruptive. One can do this unconsciously and not know it.

Try this on one case, just to check your mental axis: Give a treatment following only the lateral motions. This is not easy if your mind is midline dependent. It will not weaken the outcome at 2-3 cycles per minute and can open you to seeing the Mechanism in a different and more complete light.

Waiting for full lateral motion from the midline is a good discipline when using power points.

MAKING DECISIONS — August 21

When living with the Tide in personal decisions the following may help you, as it has helped me.

Neutral is an emptiness of will. The Tide enters this space in your heart and flows out into the world, it opens space and you follow the ease. Profound and loving events will follow.

MAKING DECISIONS — August 22

Yes is yes, it stands alone in the heart.

No is no, it stands alone in the same tensionless space. If you are neutral then nothing itself becomes a sense of direction. Nothing is something being borne. Do not be ambivalent; it will make you nervous. Wait for the heart and tell your friend, I am waiting. Maybe is never any thing worthwhile. It will always become a no.

HEALTH August 23

Neutrality ...

is a state of Health.

DEATH August 24

An elder is one who has discovered the friendship of death.

THE LONG TIDE August 25

The Long Tide is the motion of the future coming into the present.

Lesions draw force from the past.

REST August 26

If rest deepens and you are awake, its called contemplation.

FROM SHAKESPEARE August 27

There is a tide in the affairs of men

Which, taken at the flood, leads on to fortune;
Omitted, all the voyage of their life
Is bound in shallows and in miseries.
On such a full sea are we now afloat;
And we must take the current when it serves,
Or lose our ventures.[1]

1 Shakespeare, Julius Caesar Brutus, scene iii Act IV

FROM VAN DER POST

August 28

"Human beings are perhaps never more frightening than when they are convinced beyond a doubt that they are right." [1]

FROM PATANJALI

August 29

"Yogash chitta vritti nirodhah" [2]

This definition of Yoga is translated as "to still the fluctuations of the mind." W.G. Sutherland used the principle of stilling the fluid in all kinds of diseases. It is a potent anti-inflammatory and transmutative healing agent that most definitely stills the mind as the fluid comes to neutral.

When this begins to be the norm, and one is not troubled by mental-emotional traffic, then the ocean is at one's center and the virtues arise spontaneously from the Living Health.

CHANGES

August 30

Suddenly one day one senses another embryo sitting outside Zone B.

Having been intimate with the one inside, this new one is a surprise. How can this be? Then one day the outside embryo moves inside and the two embryos sit inside a circle like mirror images. The circle is Zone B. The head of one embryo touches the feet of the other; the feet of the other touch the head of the first. They form an inner circle.

Then, months later, they fuse and, as they do, a shelter is formed. The Silence becomes unbreakable.

This can happen in public places. No one will notice.

---

1 Laurens van der Post Chapter 3, Paragraph 2, The Lost World of the Kalahari.

2 Sage Patanjali, Ancient sutra

From the collection of the pieces, it is evident, that when we separate from our Health at an early age, one part of the embryo stays around us like a guardian angel, and does not return inside until we fall in love with the Health, recognizing it as our true self. Then we are safe from self-destruction and self-betrayal.

ADVICE August 31

Find the fulcrum in the event ... not in the patient.

MEETING September 1

We diagnose by what the Tide is doing.

How is the Tide guiding its power and intention. There is a wholeness to its presence.

REST September 2

Drop it all and wait....

Wait....
The attention must breathe.

MORE September 3

The Neutral, the Endpoint, and the Stillpoint are each windows into the patient's Wholeness.

The patient's unique wholeness can be appreciated at the neutral when one gets a taste of the tone, texture and tempo of the substance of the Fluid Body. At the endpoint we again see the nature of the substance of the Fluid Body and how it has changed through transmutation; we see its potential for functioning as a whole. The nature of the Stillness gives us another insight as to the nature of the patient's wholeness. Wholeness can be relative or absolute because one is evolving and growing.

ONE DAY September 4

One day, after many, many years of being her student, Ruby asked me to treat her. I was afraid. She lay supine on her bed, with her head near me at the foot of the bed. I sat and let her head rest in my hands without intention, as she had taught me. Then, she said, "treat me as if I am a newborn." Without any hesitation, I trusted her. I felt what I feel in infants. She went to sleep. The treatment was simple. I left her room in tears.

Later, I realized what she was really saying. Over and over it came back to me as a reality that must be accepted and then pursued. There is something that does not change with time—the nature of the healing forces. They are the same forever, as is the Health.

Over many years I worked to free my hands from the age of the patient.

Ruby was amazingly accurate. She got all this from Will. She was there so long with him. Today we have pediatrics courses in which we teach that you cannot treat a child as an adult, but you can treat the adult as a child. This is a reality that needs your deepest inquiry.

I am beginning to see how she helped me to think about embryonic forces being present throughout life, how she planted the seed that became Biodynamics, how she methodically worked on me so that I could see her love for the legacy from Will. She was guarding the doorway to something that words could only describe ... something that would become meaningless without a living container and active practice. Her task of helping me was full of timeliness and patience.

She was not co-dependent. If I failed she would remain neutral. If I followed, no matter how slowly, she always made me feel like I was near the finish line, because she knew the fire was too hot for a less experienced soul. She led me along, knowing I would never finish, but knew I needed to feel, at my age then, like I could come to the endpoint. She is my gold standard for an Osteopath.

FULCRUMS September 5

Fulcrums...

Fulcrums transfer the potency from cause to manifestation.

Fulcrums are in motion. They are suspended automatically shifting still points.

Fulcrums are spatially related to the midline.

A fulcrum is not a Still Point. Still Points have fulcrums.

Reciprocal tensions have fulcrums.

Attention has a fulcrum that may or may not shift.

There are moments that are fulcrums.

Fulcrums are doorways between worlds.

THE DYING PATIENT September 6

Osteopathy as stated by Dr. Still is a science of healing that sees death as a living transition.

Manipulation has nothing to offer a dying patient. Working with the Tide, however, helps a great deal.

Working with the Tide can make the transition through death healthy. Once the patient senses the Health and the love that moves through them they become peaceful and neutral to the change, sensing the future as perfect.

I have seen many patients die with an awareness of freedom and contentment. They were not all spiritual persons before they came into the realization of dying but they all felt the spiritual nature of death. Our task is to find the Health and wait.

The ego and the fear dissolve when Health is felt. One feels contentment. There is no pain. I have seen this in people who have been self-serving and mean, in people who rejected any idea of service or charity on the surface. As a general practitioner I had the privilege of seeing beyond the material view of living.

No course or mentor ever taught me to treat the dying patient. I learned it from my patients and my ignorance, always desperate to feel the Health and ask for help. It is amazingly simple, and I hope that many will learn this truth and witness what theory cannot dispense—real Osteopathy.

OSTEOPATHY — September 7

I am sometimes challenged by experts who are 'half-Osteopaths.'

"So, what is Osteopathy?" they ask expecting words that are meaningless. My answer is always the truth.

Osteopaths use their hands to engage the indwelling therapeutic forces in the patient, nothing more. No drugs, no remedies, just the indwelling gift of life. As the years have drifted by this truth has grown. I love Osteopathy the way it is. Thank God it is not more demanding of our imperfect hearts.

THE DIRECTION OF EASE — September 8

The direction of ease is the normal motion retained in the lesion field.

It is connected to every other motion inside the patient's life. One begins with a small deformed motion, and ends up inside the perfect motion in the whole organism and its environment. It is a leap of incredible proportions.

REST September 9

"Without a pause-rest between notes there could not be a musical tone."[1]

Without a Pause, there would be no awareness of the True Self moving you. Rest and Pause, and you will find the music that reminds you of Home. Home is in the pause, as the pause is a doorway.

TEACHING September 10

Teaching is what keeps an oral tradition alive.

The attitude of the teacher that makes them a real teacher is that they know what they do not know. First of all, our life span does not permit a complete knowledge of anything. Secondly, the teacher must take the student along the student's own path, not clone them. This is the only way a student can meet the Great Architect that Still speaks of. Thirdly, the goal of teaching is inquiry not political agenda. One must lead the student in the direction they are going easily.

FUNCTIONAL RESERVE September 11

Nothing ever heals by stealing energy from Peter to pay Paul.

Aggressive therapeutics can use up the reserve that heals. Our first effort is to make sure that the patient has enough power to heal. The functional reserve needs to be emphasized in our evaluation and conclusions. Does that patient have any reserve? This is our first sensory task. Listen. Where is the reserve level?

I rarely see reserve in a sick person who does not rest.

Many diets and exercise programs are depleting an already

1 Sutherland page 255 2nd edition Contribution of Thought

empty tank. Many supplements are only causing the system to burn fuel they do not have. Think about a supplement, what is it? It is a support for malnutrition in a form that often denies the true cause of the depletion. Are you taking supplements? Why? When do you address the cause behind the depletion?

Patients come in with magic formulas. I have only seen one in a thousand heal anyone, because the functional reserve is low ... low reserve cannot be cured with anything other than rest, neutrality and self-knowledge. When I work with my patients I want to know why they are taking supplements and what is behind the cause of their behavior. I ask if the supplement supports their healing or avoids the real issue of fire. I ask, "What do you want at the end of this life?" My patients listen and as they do we can slowly begin to reinstate awareness of their life. This allows their dreams to surface

What is your spiritual life like? This is a question I asked people for 50 years. It was remarkable what we all learned and did. Love is the most potent food ... it is not a supplement.

Our food today is anemic. I heard of a new organic food concentrate one can take rather than work at adequate fruit and vegetable intake. What are we doing? We are killing the instinct for material productivity. What happens to your diet when you are in full Ignition? Is there not a food we need that makes us sane? People say that this idealistic.... It is.

When do we live in the motion towards normal that drives us into eternity and rest? What fills up the tank? Fire ... fire from where?

Still believed, and proved, that God's drugstore is inside us.

Cause and effect are an over-simplification of reality.

Just as reductionism and superficiality have overtaken our training, cause and effect is a trap. Dr. Still pointed us away from the trap of cause and effect by pointing us towards Cause on another level.

Look at the message of Laurens van der Post:

It is the not-yet in the now
The taste of a fruit that does not yet exist
Hanging the blossom on the bough.[1]

Between cause……………….and……………….effect is a third element of action. The 'not-yet' in the present, something that is active in the true relationship of what seems to be happening but is not happening the way it appears in linear thinking.

One manner of seeing into cause and effect more clearly is to add this third element to the action of what appears to be cause and effect—the 'not-yet.' Cause and effect are not as real as one's mind suggests. For example, I am sick ... I ate bad food ... seems real enough, but what else is in the story that makes it deeper?

I am aiming at the reality that exists in patients … the reality that we are supposed to realize in order help them. It is not in the linear cause and effect picture. You can actually feel something other in the laws as you witness them.

Let's ponder this by sensation as we live and treat, let's look again for a greater geometry than cause and effect.

1 Laurens van der Post page 54 Venture to the Interior

EMBRYOLOGY September 13

According to Blechschmidt, the science of embryology states that the entire blueprint of a being exists from conception.

It unfolds from a mysterious silent clock. This unfoldment is an after effect of complete wholeness. We do not generally appreciate that we are done before we begin, that we do not become whole as we grow. Osteopathy is like this. Something moves us towards completion. We call this image behind the scene the Health. It is not docile … it is the equation of existence.

LAURENS van der POST September 14

"It is as if one incorporates within one's own being all the time that has ever been and can ever be, and that fever is either the vehicle itself or evidence of the means by which one is forced from one time context into another. The moment one's fever rises from normal one's self ceases to be contemporary.

I have emerged from serious illness with the conviction of having been in a time anterior to the present. The feeling has persisted despite my failure to define it …. our battle for survival is fought out at a level and in a spirit of which we have little consciousness."[1]

Laurens van der Post was an explorer of the first man. The African Bushman, the noblest of all human tribes, was his life's role model of this first man in all of us. The Bushmen of Africa were exterminated by both white and black Africans. Mr. Van der Post was a dear friend of both Carl Jung and Helen Luke. His writings are very beautiful. He wished for us all to sense a deeper functioning being hidden in the darkness of our soul, something that was fully in the image of Harmony.

1 Laurens van der Post page 105 Venture to the Interior

LONG-TIDE September 15

"......while the day spilled like a tidal wave over the horizon."[1]

REST September 16

Rest.................................as you rest, watch your breathing and the breathing of the Sea Around you.[2]

INVOLUNTARY BRAIN MOTIONS September 17

Imagine discovering all that Sutherland wrote about in The Tour of the Minnow.[3]

I had the privilege of attending a closed meeting sponsored by the Cranial Academy between four Osteopaths and two researchers, one from Russia and one from The Chicago School of Medicine. Both men were researching slow cranial rhythms. The problem they faced with their research was how to the filter out the motion generated in the brain from heart pulsations and thoracic respiration. As I listened to their dilemma, I thought, "How amazing is the human brain? We as observers can filter out whatever we wish and focus on selected details." This is how Sutherland was able to retrieve information that instruments find obscure. All of a sudden the science of Osteopathy seemed much more accurate than laboratory science. Of course, I kept this to myself but those who ridicule Sutherland and his followers are uneducated about observation, and the human brain, and how amazing its perceptional function is.

Eventually, many years after Sutherland perceived, described, and taught about it, both scientists documented the response of the brain to the Long-Tide in a complex manner. Then the scientists wanted to feel the slow rates with their hands.

1 Laurens van der Post page 75 Venture to the Interior
2 see Bibliography and Notes
3 Sutherland page 346 2nd edition Contributions of Thought

We did a practical with them. They had the discipline and objectivity to follow and succeed. It was a wonderful few days. For some reason no report was ever published by the Academy.

BUOYANCY September 18

When one evaluates the CNS, this picture is the basic picture of normal

The brain floats. It has fluid inside, outside and through it. Imagine for a moment this tadpole-like living function ... suspended by fluid: fluid in the neural tube, fluid in the cisterns and fluid within the brain itself. There is fluid flowing in and out. It is a floating automatically shifting organ. Besides these fluids, we have the fluid body itself, as an anti-gravitational sustaining force. The fluid body creates the brain and can repair it. All of these fluids suspend and float the tadpole. If everything is normal, the whole CNS moves in relationship to the midline and a suspended fulcrum at lamina terminalis. The fluid motion is synchronized with the motion of the tissue of the brain, which spirals or coils along its developmental pathway. It does this during the inhalation phase and there is an accompanying longitudinal fluctuation, which rises up from the coccyx to the lamina terminalis, arriving there at the extreme end of the inhalation phase of primary respiration at 2 to 3 cycles per minute. All this timing and synchronization is from the Health, which tries to move all function towards the original blueprint. The potency that drives the mechanism is likewise transmutating any resistance towards a harmonic re-intergration of the parts to the whole and normalizing function.

I have done thousands of consults for my colleagues ... the most common thing I find is a lack of diagnostic precision. It seems that people want to get into the lesion and fix it rather than put it in perspective within the whole.

GROWTH September 19

The process of growth unfolds from the Health.

There is no structure, only form arising and dying. When growth stops one's function and form become repetitive and adynamic.

THORACIC RESPIRATION September 20

Thoracic Respiration does not make an impression within the fluid body in most adults.

In children, it suffuses the fluid body and brings the potency of Thoracic and Primary Respiration into a single Potency that transmutes the past and forms the future.

What can this mean?

THORACIC RESPIRATION September 21

In children, there is one breathing expression from a single fulcrum.

Thoracic and Primary Respiration are expressing themselves from one point or origin, with different formats.

What does this mean?

When children are isolated from the family circle, Thoracic Respiration desynchronizes and establishes a fulcrum separate from Primary Respiration. We see this when children have been in the hospital, or have had surgery, even though the parents sleep there. Surgery most often causes a shift from one to multiple fulcrums. When the breathings separate from each other, the mothers notice the eyes of their child have become dull. We need to be alert to the oneness of breathing in children. If it is broken then the treatment is simple. Synchronize with the pattern of Thoracic Respiration during its inhalation period. This will often successfully return the unity of breathing in a child.

INVOLUNTARY MOTION

September 22

The involuntary motion of the sacrum and coccyx need to be highlighted in any evaluation of the spine. The motion occurs in response to Thoracic Respiration and is vital to long term health of the bony elements but also the meninges. The prevention of spinal stenosis depends on this motion between the Thoracic Respiration and the sacral-coccygeal area.

The physiological motion of the dura is dependent on this motion. It is an anti-inflammatory movement. This is so overlooked that it bewilders me when I find out how little attention is paid to this truth. Additionally, the motion in these elements, as an effect of Primary Respiration, is vital to the physiological momentum of the tissues of all levels. The vertical rise, with inhalation towards lamina terminalis, of this whole area is an elemental movement necessary for the healthy function of the bones, discs, and meninges. Please reflect upon this and incorporate this into your thinking.

REST

September 23

Wait in the Meeting Place.

Rest without expectation. You will be met and healed.

CHARLIE September 24

Charlie came to see me because of a herniated disc.

He was earthy, clear and honest. He looked like an unkept room but his appearance was a decoy for an intelligent and loving soul.

As I treated him, I noticed a scar on his left forearm. I inquired about it. Charlie said "That was a big black growth, about the size of a quarter. The doctor took it off. He wanted me to take drugs to cure the metastasis; I was not interested. The doctor said I could die." He had had a malignant melanoma. There was a long pause of several minutes, the air deepened. I could feel the Tide surround us, as it often does when secrets are unfolding. He continued. "I told that doctor, 'what do you know about death and life?'" Then Charlie said to me "I have seen what you can not even imagine. I was in Vietnam. When I arrived and stepped ashore there was a pick-up truck full of dead children that passed in front of me. So, what do you know about life and death?" Charlie then told me he just walked out of that doctor's office never to return.

There was a lot of wisdom in Charlie, great wisdom. He honored me by trusting me. He said he had never told anyone before ... this was 25 years later. The melanoma never bothered him; he was now ten years from the excision. Charlie drank a lot, worked hard and fell in love one summer late in his years. He had seen man's inhumanity in a way I was frightened to envision.

I have never felt so privileged to hold another man's secret.

CLEM September 25

Clem was a retired Major.

He was a big tall guy with a commanding voice and presence. I was young, maybe thirty-three. He came in all bent over. He had been lying on the floor for a week with sciatica. I gave him a treatment using the involuntary motion present in the lesion. It was maybe twelve minutes. As I finished and said I

was done, He said, 'This is bullshit!'
He was forceful but I could understand his point of view. "O.K.", I said, "I will make you a deal. If you become no better, there is no charge. But, if you are better, then you pay double … how's that?" He grumbled and left without comment.

Two days later I called to check on him, as I usually do. He answered the phone. I said who was calling. There was silence. 'I am really well', he said. I was happy for him and told him to check in with me in a week for some fine-tuning. As I went to hang up the phone he said, "Wait! I want to bring my wife." Clem and his wife became longtime patients who always had a joke about my 'voodoo'.… He lived well past ninety.

I do not charge patients who do not benefit from my efforts.

DR. ANNE WALES ON ACUTE ILLNESS September 26

Disease is a process of getting well.

Disease is a process in the whole patient.

We diagnose by getting into the body and thinking, feeling, and knowing, not by deductive reasoning.

Good care begins at the end of an acute illness. We are interested in cause.

What makes disease self-limiting?

What does connective tissue have to do with acute illness?

What happens in the extra-cellular space, the membrane of the cell, and the intracellular space during acute illness?

What makes lymphocytes migrate to the site of need?

Breathing is a lymphatic pump!

What generates fever? Where does the energy come from?

Optimize lymphatic flow!

DR. ANNE WALES — September 27

The bones are the handles for access to the body ...

We begin with connective tissue (mesenchyme) and proceed.

The body is self-regulating, self-correcting, and self-healing.

Osteopathy's earliest conquest was in pulmonary disease during the 1928 influenza epidemic, not in treating musculoskeletal disease.

What monitors the anatomical-physiological pattern, what model does it use for normal?

Does anything see the whole body simultaneously?

Get at where the body is trying to solve the problem, do not diagnose!

What does the body do when it reaches normal?

How well is your patient?

Fortunately, patients are not limited to one doctor.

THE SCALES — September 28

All of my mentors who were with Will loved to talk about the story of the Balance Scales.

Will was in a country store in Cape Cod. He saw an old set of balance scales hanging from the ceiling. He talked about the fulcrum through which balance worked ... a stillpoint, the point of power for the function of the scales—a fulcrum. It hardly took a touch to shift it, he said. As he was explaining this to those with him, the wind came through the doorway and the scales shifted. He was delighted.[1]

---

1 Sutherland page 346 2nd edition Contributions of Thought

This metaphor is not a metaphor. The reality of this is so sweet that it must be taught as a basic skill and a natural state of being.

I heard this story often and it still has more in it than the last time it was told!

NEW BEGINNINGS — September 29

In 1991 Anne wrote a reply to a letter I sent her. She sent a picture of Will Sutherland and said, "It shows his spirit." She also wrote: "my last conversation with Will was in the spring of 1954. I asked him what accounts for the fluctuation of the CSF in its natural cavity and he said he did not know."

Can we follow his humility and fearlessness and let our model, die, as he did?

Can we think independent of what we know?

REST — September 30

Suffused rest is a spontaneous effect of the Health.

SAVING FOR A RAINY DAY — October 1

Keep a journal of all the intercessions by the Tide.

Record all those moments of beauty and healing that come into your day. When it rains, read your book. Do not keep any other information in this journal ... it is spiritual, not psychological or technical. This will keep your rainy days brief. I am sure you have noticed how memory of many great events is overshadowed by one small insult ... the truth buried by one tiny challenge. This is a curious thing. The journal can help. As your memory of the truth enters the foreground, the challenges will not shift your state away from the Tide.

B.L.T. October 2

Balanced ligamentous tension is about the ligaments.

Dr. Wales said many times that people are feeling the bones when they should be just balancing the ligamentous tension and letting that allow the bones to move. There is no direct contact with bone during B.L.T. This is not an easy task and if you are a teacher know that your students need to practice this in order to understand the deeper realities in these principles.

Do not rush by this milestone.

MORE THAN ONE October 3

"You are not the last station on the railway, doctor!"

When I was disappointed in my skill and was not able to help someone as I believed I should, Ruby would remind me that we are not the end all.

ROLLIN October 4

"If you are only aware of the head, you are limited."[1]

I am so grateful to Rollin for his help from 1966 until he retired. He was very clear about perception, so I will begin there. Wherever you are on the body, there must be no attention directed to the part. Listen from wherever you are with a capitol L. The key is using the attention to Listen not focusing one's intention on the part. This change in perception will take years. Then all there is is wholeness and the Tide.

1 See Bibliography and Notes

ROLLIN October 5

If the patient is trying to steal energy, I contact my silent space and then the patient's.

Just recognize … realize what is going on … do not analyze … just your Mechanism in touch with the patients Mechanism. No personality, no ego, just two … in contact with one place. When I meditate with God, again its one to one, nothing in between.[1]

Rollin clearly is not hiding. Neutrality is an aspect of the Health and Divinity. So he did not hide from negative forces he was naturally safe where he was.

He was, I believe, pointing towards neutrality in the observer. He moves to the Health in himself and the patient, which is untouchable by negative forces.

ROLLIN October 6

Don't anticipate.[2]

REST October 7

When you get a pause in a treatment make sure you let your attention retreat from the therapeutic activity.
Rest.
The pauses are very important.

1 See Bibliography and Notes
2 See Bibliography and Notes

STUDY SOME MORE October 8

Sutherland noted that lesions were positional exaggerations.

He then noted that the lesion had motion in the direction of insult. The direction of ease is often in the same direction as the positional exaggerations. This teaching is biomechanical, as are the patterns that one sees from using this model. Then comes the fluid model teachings; the fluid lesions too. The fluid lesion does not match the biomechanical pattern.

Now we see the dilemma of technique applied with force … but wait … the fluid in the fluid can lesion too. Now we have perhaps three patterns to discern but also the loss to power in the whole.

Now what does one do?

Sutherland suggests holding the tissue and the fluid fluctuation at the balance point. Then you will feel a tug.[1]

Later, he stops holding….

See if you can follow the path he took … your students will follow his pattern too because the mind needs to change it's orientation.

REVIEW OVER AND OVER October 9

Thoracic Respiration in adults is 6 seconds per cycle, when in neutral. Primary respiration is poly-rhythmic at 24 seconds per cycle, and 100 seconds per cycle. They are related by a factor of four.

Sutherland stated that if "all the fulcrums were synchronized there would be peace and harmony"[2]. One can easily see that the there could be a balance point for all of these cycles … if

1 Sutherland Page 349 2nd Edition Contributions of Thought see Bibliography and Notes
2 Sutherland See Bibliography and Notes

the perception was unwavering with the circumstances.

When this happens for a beginner, it is usually a synchronization that occurs at the peak of inhalation, after 24 seconds, when Thoracic Respiration goes into a deep inhalation during the groundswell of the therapeutics in the fluid body. The groundswell is an extra large wave of inhalation that heralds disengagement in the whole.[1]

When full synchronization occurs the rates end because there is only one fulcrum … all we perceive is time passing and eternal Stillness.

This is natural augmentation not framed by human force.

SOMETIMES WE TWITCH — October 10

Study diodes.

Sometimes the operator's hands twitch. When the electric forces in the inertia release it should be unnoticeable. If we hold the lesion field without being neutral the energy discharged from the lesion can enter us, unless there is an instinctive twitch to prevent the energy from coming into us. We are shaking it off before it enters … this is not a conscious act; it is instinct.

Dr. Fulford would have us ground our systems after a treatment to remove any excess energy … he would grab a faucet in the sink and let the energy go back to the earth. Triple yarrow tincture helps too.

I have found over time that all the need for these efforts has passed.

1 See Bibliography and Notes

LESIONS

October 11

Fluid lesions are not symmetrical unless they are iatrogenic.

When you come across beautiful lesions, ones that are perfect forms … reflect, look again, are the shapes part of the whole or are they isolated like islands of different tone. These beautifully shaped lesions are imprints from a treatment that was done to the patient. They are iatrogenic lesions. Treat the iatrogenic lesion as you would any other insult that needs rebalancing.

The opposite effect occurs also. Some twenty years after Ruby Day treated someone, I could feel the connection, in the patient, with the Health, from her work. This form of integration and connection shows Ruby's artistry and skill in working with the Health.

LESIONS

October 12

Fluid fluctuations that reveal no connection to a midline are lesions.

In Health, the connection a fluid has with the midline reveals a therapeutic wave that will retreat after a few moments or minutes.

EV4

October 13

EV4 is a language created for the Biodynamic curriculum.

It is not a technique. It either occurs spontaneously or it is a direction of ease that one can follow without giving it a direction. Unfortunately, I have been misquoted in all the writings I am aware of, and force is always added as the language of EV4 is changed to technique … why do we need force? Why do people insist on it?

REST October 14

Resting before you are tired creates a life.

You enter into the domain of third level stillness for the intensity of companionship.

EV4 AND CV4 ARE THE SAME PRINCIPLE October 15

Even today 20 years after Sutherland first taught it, there are still operators working the bones to center the fluid in the fluid. The goal of CV4 and EV4 is the same. They both bring the fluid body to neutral or idling so that the Longitudinal Fluctuation can be reestablished to provide the power and spatial dynamics to heal and renew the fluid body as a whole. Direct action is not, necessary. Leave the bones alone, unless the patient has a perfect head!

Sutherland was very adept at getting Thoracic Respiration to neutral — an art of extreme precision. He eventually found his method for getting neutral in the fluid body ... he actually says that the bones do not need to be addressed.

Bring the fluid in the fluid in the direction of ease and it will go to neutral. This is a central principle in Osteopathy as Still and Sutherland taught it: finding neutral.

There is more than meets the eye, much more.

I hope you know the Sutherland fulcrum. If not, read everything written about it in all of Sutherland's writings before you proceed.

At the cephalic end of the notochord just under the Lamina Terminalis and the Diaphragm Sellae at the junction of the Pre and Post Sphenoid is a point of major importance. We call it the tip of the notochord but in fact the notochord ends at this point. This point is the geometric place of organization of the development of the CNS.

Movements from this point or fulcrum unfold like a plant from a seed. The Sutherland Fulcrum begins here and, as the intracranial development occurs, the fulcrum moves from this point of origin in an anterior, superior, posterior and inferior motion. This curve or spiral motion carries potency as well as fluid and tissue. It carries the power from the point of origin to the posterior cranial fossa. The point becomes the Sutherland Fulcrum. The fulcrum is potency and as it leaves the center to reside at the periphery it remains connected along the spiral pathway of its journey to the central axis of growth and development.

Once in its final position it lies on a diagonal with the central point of origin at the tip of the notochord - the central fulcrum for the whole cranium. This diagonal is a line of potency that unites the fulcrum with the ignition system.

The journey from the center to the periphery is not finished at birth. It takes 28 years to complete the wholeness of an embryonic journey.

The Sutherland Fulcrum is not the anatomic center of the dural system; the Diaphragm Sellae, and more specifically a doorway at the center of the Diaphragm Sellae just above the tip of the notochord, is the anatomic center.

So, think about these lines and the points and see what you learn.

THE MIDLINE

October 17

The Midline centers us.

This is how we know we are at the midline of the functions for Zone B ... it centers us when we approach it. The midline in this context is a doorway to the ocean of Dynamic Stillness that becomes the Meeting Place where the Master appears once we are at home with being neutral.

The sensation that overshadows us is that we are will-less and
held safely in emptiness, ready for being healed....
Then something comes and transmutes the senses.

THE CONTINUUM

October 18

"If the cerebrospinal fluid locks down on the olfactory bulbs the motion of the ethmoid is locked."[1]

This fact from Sutherland when processed raises some question about the real nature of an osteopathic lesion. Try and explain how this happens.

THE CONTINUUM

October 19

"Release the articular mechanism and a fluid lift of the cerebellum corrects the situation."[2]

How is this possible?

1 Sutherland Page 350 2nd edition of Contributions of Thought.
2 Sutherland page 350 2nd Edition Contributions of Thought

DIAGNOSTICS October 20

Do you discern the difference between the following circumstances:

- An Osteopathic lesion
- A sub-luxation
- A metabolic lesion
- Intra-membranous shears
- Intra-osseous lesions originating in fluid restrictions
- The layers of the C.N.S. and the location of the primary area of need
- Iatrogenic lesions induced by you while you are working or by someone before you
- Your conscience and your desire
- Fluid body lesions
- Projections

Can you tell which of these is present by sensing?

REST October 21

There is a somatic sensation of eternity. Rest and it will find you.

THE FULCRUM October 22

"The fulcrum point, the still point in the fluctuation of the cerebrospinal fluid where you come close in your understanding of .... the "highest known element."

What does Sutherland mean by this? He is using Still's principle of the "highest known element." This is about the ultimate Potency that can heal disease. Still associated it with the "River of Life"[1] that irrigates the "withering fields"[2] and restores normal physiological flow. When one comes to this level of stillness it is not in the patient but through everything.

1 Still page 39 Philosophy of Osteopathy
2 Still page 39 Philosophy of Osteopathy See Bibliography and Notes

Flowing through the stillness is the "River of Life." These are not words but a living reality. It cannot be seen if one is doing the treatment with any force. Unfortunately, most CV4 do not access this reality because of the technique employed. One cannot read Still and Sutherland clearly unless one understands the words and Still's intention. "The River of Life" is not a philosophical term; it is supernatural and from God's outpouring of creation. It will create healing that is beyond the assumptive mind.

THIRD LEVEL STILLNESS October 23

I want you to understand that this work takes time and real inner sacrifices.

To see into the "Laws not framed by human hands"[1] is not easy. People are abusing this work by thinking they know—moving into a reality that they do not appreciate except as an idea. Real Osteopathy is challenging; it requires some inner changes that are severe.

Third level stillness is such a place. Draw a circle. The black line of the circle is the outer edge of third level stillness. The substance in the circle is what you will experience once you are at the outer edge; inside the circle is a world we do not transcend with our power and will.

Having traversed the whole landscape several things happen: one, you wait in neutrality, two, you rest beyond the ego's desire for existence, three, you are met by a Living Presence that touches you and as a result of that touch you are transmutated into a person that surprises even you. This new person is a gift from the Master ... you cannot own it. Then four, you begin to see a new world through the eyes of the Master. You are not at a distance from Him, you are with Him and see what He sees the way He sees it.

This is not an experience; it is a relationship of dependency

1 Sutherland page 300 and 307 2nd edition Contribution of Thought also See Bibliography and Notes

and deep child-like love for the Creation that moves through Life. The world of third level stillness opens only when you have the key and know the Master is your beloved teacher and saving grace ... period.

I hear a lot of talk about being in the third level.... Be careful you are not being clever.

The death of the observer is a hard and long journey ... do not assume and loose the potential of finding the wholeness in Health.

This is a warning to not get lost and end up with nothing but a great grieving heart.

THE LOSS OF A COMMUNITY — October 24

There are three defections from the truth of Osteopathy.

The worst is the idea of a musculo-skeletal specialist, the next is the illusion of M.D. equality, rather than a unique profession and the third is the 'new age' lack of boundaries and discipline. All these influences are killing the profession.

Osteopathy cannot be placed outside of itself. Renaming the manual skills Neuro-musculoskeltal Medicine as a separate specialty or branch of practice is a deep betrayal of Osteopathy as a science.

Proclaiming that the training of a doctor of Osteopathy and a medical doctor is identical, in an effort to obtain a higher or equal status to M.D.'s, is an ironic fallacy. I am amazed at how easy people assume our profession is, when in fact it requires more knowledge and training than an M.D's.

Be careful of experts who believe they understand Osteopathy. Why should they anyway? They have never practiced Osteopathy or studied with Sutherland or his students. To practice Osteopathy is not anything like what I have been told by cranio-sacral therapists that they do. I have witnessed this deception: non-Osteopathic persons taking Osteopathic ideas and presenting themselves as teachers of this work. I have met some of these people and they do not understand Osteopathy in any form but their own imaginings; they often believe that they understand what the great ones have said. The great ones were great because of their teachers and the authority given them by a legacy that is strenuous.

We need to reclaim our community or accept the death of Osteopathy.

QUESTION October 25

Why does the power and influence of Thoracic Respiration increase as the breath idles and becomes smaller?

TRUTH October 26

The body knows its Creator.

Not Zone A, but the body without the ego's influence.... Again we come to one ultimate Osteopathic question what is it like to be normal?

ADD ON October 27

Do you add compression to a lesion with motion?

Why? When? How?
Have we forgotten that all lesions have motion that is present?
otherwise they would necrose ...would they not?
So why add on?

REST October 28

Dr. Sutherland recommended that we read Hilton's book on Rest and Pain.[1]

CENTERING October 29

Sometimes we hold the center.

When centering for any reason, check and see if you are holding the space in which the centering occurs. The space where you center yourself should be free to move in and out and around as it intends. It is enlightening to see oneself confining the center from automatically shifting. Let the center hold you as it did when you were made.

ORIENTATION October 30

Early in our meetings, Ruby Day told me the following:

The whole thoracic spine can be treated as a single vertebra. Having one's hands at the two ends, one engages motion in the whole region as one event. Then one synchronizes and the whole column disengages. She said it coils and uncoils like a snake. This was from Will.[2]

THE TIDE October 31

The word Tide and the word tide
express two different ideas of potency.

One is absolute the other relative. One can be directed by human hands the other cannot. The Tide is more intelligent than the brain, which it creates. The tide is a fluid in the fluid. The Tide directly transmutates a pattern of disease through the entire body ... simultaneously!

---

1 See Bibliography of Contributions of thought.
2 See Bibliography and Notes

TEMPO November 1

The unfolding of therapeutic changes must fit into the tempo of the whole, as it is already engaged, before treatment is administered.

One can learn to be aware of what is already happening before engaging new therapeutics; this knowledge potentiates the treatment. This avoids superimposing a new pattern on the whole which has a tempo. Otherwise the Tide has to rebalance the part into the Whole.

EXPLORERS November 2

Both Carl Jung and William Sutherland went so far into the unknown that they did not know, at times, if they would regain their footing.

They did not know if they would get back to their realty without severe damage to themselves. Men like this understand something that onlookers will never appreciate. Think about going beyond your knowledge with out any sense of self-preservation. To read and believe one comprehends is a small drop compared to going beyond one's absolute limit.

FAITH November 3

St. Francis, in one day, lived a decision to be a different being. Then came the miracles!

REST November 4

What is the quality of the effect of resting?

Could we say that conscious rest brings one home?

TRUST November 5

Trusting in the unknown.

Trusting the Tide.
Trusting the unseen, the not-yet.
Trusting the eternal.
All this is not going to feel safe. It is an abyss that one must endure, or not.

THE TIDE November 6

No force is necessary, not even intention.

THE TIDE November 7

The Tide is not the waves moving in the fluid. It is what moves the waves, shapes them, and directs them.

CENTERING November 8

There are many degrees of centering, many kinds and methods.

The method we engage is contemplation, entering an interior place of silence and emptiness. This place is found in ourselves after much discipline and service.

Once you have entered the silent room, where thoughts end and being begins, notice the boundary of the center ... is it free? Or are you unconsciously holding it? Are you in a place of escape? Let the center flow ... as it wishes. This begins to create motion where the Tide can flow out of you into the world without restriction. This is called Dynamic Centering in our work because it allows the Dynamic Stillness to move and that will lead to many peaceful consequences for us all.

GROWTH

November 9

Wholeness moves; this gives the appearance of the parts moving.

It is like embryonic Thai Chi. This is how we all heal, in spite of our need to explain change in ourselves as improvement in the parts. We miss the changing action of wholeness.

BEGIN

November 10

Always begin with the Health!

This means ultimately to find Beauty. Find it in the moment you are in.... This may not be 'in' the patient. Find something that makes you peaceful, joyful. This is the Health.

REST

November 11

One pauses ....

A rest between the thoughts ... between the senses ...
Between inhalation and exhalation
A doorway leads to a Dynamic Stillness
That leads to endless Space ...
That leads to the end of knowing ...
That leads to the Master.
That leads to the Health.

HANDS

November 12

Always look up with your hands ... no matter how they are positioned.

This will reveal a great change in your perception.

IMAGINE November 13

The Tide is a living presence; it is not just energy.

How can this be?
It enters our awareness in such limited ways.
Think....

It provides Fire/ Transmutations/ Form/ Limits/ Function/ Healing/ Wisdom/ Rates/ Shifts/ Neutrals/ Pause/ Still points/ Stillness/ Compensation/ Breathing/ Love....

What is the Tide in its Wholeness?

ENERGY November 14

In the West this idea is an escape from surrendering will and being intimate with LIFE.

LOVE November 15

If we are at peace with our own stink we can love others.

Otherwise we will not see the common wound we all live in.

VECTORS November 16

Sutherland mentions the capacity of fluid to lesion tissue function.

Traumatic forces that enter the posterior cranial fossa and upper cervicals are not held there. The insults move forward into the middle face. If we always look at the tissue in the cranial vertebral junction for resolution we will miss lesion fulcrums in the middle face fluid field. This, in fact, is where we find most of the inertia for the whole lesion. Release of the fluid field releases the entire lesion including the tissue restrictions in the posterior head and neck.

Also, trauma to the dental arches may produce a vector that locks up the fluid at Lambda. This feels odd - like a second tent, or that the tent is too high, when it is not.

THE RESPIRATORY SINUS November 17

There are not separate sinuses in the head.

They are one. The different names confuse the underlying reality. There is only one sinus that branches. Check the embryology of this and you will see one of the limits anatomists introduce into the clinical sense we develop of function. The same limits are introduced by the biomechanical model of the sinuses. Many want the facts. The fact is the whole sinus is a unit not several separate sinuses

REST November 18

To hold a palatine ...

... weightless with grace, delicately formed like a perfect petal, a window into heaven, one does not think of gears but rather the precision of the Architect. We can memorize the planes and angles and miss such refinery. Rest in the beauty of wholeness. Herein is the Tide.

We have a choice to make.

HANDS November 19

Be careful ...

Both hands should feel the whole. If one hand feels the left side and one the right side there will be a false midline created. Practice using one hand to feel the whole, then the other.

VERTICAL HEIGHT — November 20

This activity is in the wholeness.

Imagine the odontoid, the mandible, the clivus, the mastoid process, the styloid process, the teeth, the sternum, the abdomen, the pelvis, and the legs all being elongated as a single event.

STATES AND RATES — November 21

The scheme of things:

Rate: 8-14 cycles/minute — Mental state: fluctuates, lots of ideas, thoughts and distractions

Rate: 2-3 cycles/minute — Mental state: mental pauses, thoughts range into more order

Rate: 100 seconds/cycle — Mental state: Aware of the horizon and all that moves in Nature.

Rate: Dynamic Stillness—Mental state: Stillness fills Zone D. The movement of the long-tide is not present. This is called third level stillness. It empties the mind and prepares it for conversion by the Master.

Rate: Breath of Life—The movement of Eternity, Creation and Love suffuse all. The sense of I is lost. All of life is one movement.

WHOLENESS — November 22

Wholeness is not altered by disease.

GLASS HOUSE

November 23

The House Under the Sea[1] is like glass ... the sea is luminous.

The House is transparent to the light ... it passes through undiminished.
Feel the transparency of the soma.

OSTEOPATHY

November 24

Osteopathy was discovered by Dr. Still.

He did not claim to have created it. He came to understand that Osteopathy is a word used to describe natural laws placed into human beings before they were born. These laws, known and unknown, are what we call Osteopathy. The goal of an Osteopathic education is to give us the tools to perceive these innate laws and appreciate the plumb-line which is what one calls conscience in spiritual traditions. Conscience is a knowing that proceeds from the discernment of the Health in any living or non-living element. Osteopathy was before Still ... and the Teacher we seek is in this Eternity.

REST

November 25

.... This means .... Which means ... Stop thinking.... Pause ... and rest.... Even in the conversation or while reading.

Do you get the point?

1 See Bibliography and Notes

FIRE November 26

Primary Respiration expresses involuntary motion.

One should note the tone, texture, shape and tempo of the inhalation phase and the exhalation phase at different rates and at different potencies. Familiarity with these natural and divine laws will bring one closer to communication. Knowing this allows our understanding of the individual patient to be more accurate.

FIRE November 27

The tone and texture of the shape of the inhalation and exhalation phases is not a mechanically induced breathing. It is not like a bellows. Think what is making the shape of the breath as it moves?

The shape is created by the Potency of the Tide … which is Fire.

FIRE November 28

Fire is not the fire one experiences when one lights a match.

The fire of Primary Respiration transmutates without wounding us. What is the nature of this kind of Fire? It inscribes a shape as it burns. As the old is burned away, as it is transmutated, a space is created; the space has shape. It is somewhat similar to a grass fire that leaves a shape behind its burning. Shape itself, in human forms, is a result of the Wisdom of fire. It comes from a Biodynamic process.

FIRE November 29

The tone, texture, and tempo of the transmutation are related to the substance of that being burned; that is, the nature of the lesion.

WILL

November 30

Rollin Becker said to me, "The treatment begins when the will of the patient surrenders to the will of the Tide."[1]

Waiting for this is necessary.

MECHANICAL FULCRUMS

December 1

The artistry of biomechanical methods is rarely seen anymore.

It is as precise as one can imagine. The force needed is proportionate to the skill of the operator: less force is required when there is more skill, because the operator can apply it through a small balance point - the fulcrum. More force is needed when one is trying the override the barrier in the lesion without first finding a balance point of suspension for the tissue forces.

The fulcrum is searched for quietly without disturbing the autonomic nervous system. It is as small as a pencil dot. Once the lesion is suspended on the fulcrum the thrust is simple and easy.

This principle can be applied in many circumstances.

REST

December 2

Third Level Stillness is called the Dynamic Stillness.

It centers us. We begin occasionally to feel a neutral that has no connection to our personal will. It holds us on its center. Here we enter a House under the Sea. [2]We are a guest. We rest.[3]

---

1 See Bibliography and Notes
2 See Bibliography and Notes
3 Jim Jealous page 50 Pediatrics 1 Manual,

ATTENTION FLOWS — December 3

Distraction occurs when the attention flows outwards away from oneself into an event.

The event can be our projection or something outside us in the immediate environment. The attention sticks to the phenomena and is absorbed continuously.

When attention flows inwardly it becomes remarkably quieting and healing inside, but only if it continues to flow—to live. If the attention goes inwards and stops in the head one begins thinking in an unfocused manner.

If it flows inwards and stops in the heart one becomes self centered and emotions rule ones self expression. Deeper in the Heart is the whole, an emptiness that the creator fills with fire.

Direct the attention inwards within yourself ... let it flow ... many truths will be seen. If you wish to love there will be a doorway that opens.

FULCRUMS — December 4

The fulcrum for the whole is the Whole.

This requires some meditation. It sounds good but do you understand the consequences of this experience as your only reality?

SELF-IMAGE — December 5

Our true image is the embryo.

Contact this sweet innocence and your mask will begin to fade.....fall in love with this image... see it in your patients and yourself.

NEUTRAL December 6

"When matter ceases to be divisible .... it becomes a fluid of life ...

... and easily unites with other atoms and is a mass or body of living matter and re-crystallizes into the form given by parent causes."[1]

Dr. Still points us to the Fluid Body. What do you think he means by an indivisible matter?

FROM A LETTER RECEIVED IN 1995 December 7

"We live in a world of dimension but we come from non-dimension."[2]

I have been thinking, over the past few months, about the nature of the stillpoint and how it transforms.

At the point of balanced tension, be it fluid or tissue, all forces are balanced about a point; a place of non-dimension. It feels like a window into another world ... a world which is in resonance with the world of non-dimension. At this moment there is an opportunity for the primordial nature of what we are to manifest through that non-dimensional window and transform directly, side-stepping the ordinary process of somatization or conditioned attitudes and emotional patterns that are the product of the past. It is an opportunity for the not-yet to be expressed purely in all its freshness. This fluid stillness that envelopes the world in its process of manifestation, this love that permeates our world, does not seem interested in the virtues of the practitioner or the patient, except that it requires stillness for all the waves to be gathered into one force.

1 Still, pages 254-255The philosophy and Mechanical Principles
2 Rumi 1207 – 17 December 1273

STILLNESS IS NOT STILL — December 8

Stillness ripens the fruit.

The fruit opens. The seeds drops. It germinates. There is a new sensorium. A new world where the purpose of life is Life ... the beautiful incarnation of Divine Love flowing, changing ... Eternally.

Stillness may seem motionless. It is often stated to be an end in itself as if Stillness was a place of completion - it is not. Stillness is a place of conversion, of transmutation. Herein is the domain where the observer can die and rise up closer to Originality.

The observer who senses stillness needs to be neutral to the stillness, to rest ... and wait for the breathing and the Master and the healing and the end of the known. Stillness is a meeting place a room in a house where we wait in peace. Many years are passed here.

There is a death that stillness creates. We die to awaken in a new way... only to find more to become. To die ... at the hands of Love is what Stillness prepares us for.

REST — December 9

We have inner senses and outer senses.

The inner senses have been suppressed. The inner sense of smell is the intuitive understanding of a moment. The inner sense of taste is conscience. The inner sense of sight is a vision. The inner sense of hearing understands the pauses. The inner sense of touch is awake only to the flow of love. These inner senses operate at a deeper and more integrated level than the cultured senses. As a matter of fact, the two kinds of senses are often in contradiction. This can lead to continued ambivalence about life.

To hear the inner senses the rational mind must be quiet. We must pause.

VISION

December 10

Illusion: Feeds the ego, projections outward and inward are lesions.

Natural Vision: The horizon, the sea around us.

Inner Vision: The heart, the light of fire, the void, another breath.

Emptiness: Blindness occurs. The wounded senses die.

Inspired Vision: the senses are converted by the Master, the Health appears; sight is given.

One eye: Love suffuses and creates the content of the moment.

SIT

December 11

Sit ... watch ... sit and observe

... then realize that the observer has many levels and must always die on one level to be discerning on another new level. Let the observer seek its own death ... because Love is asking us to come closer.

SKILL

December 12

New skill makes us feel naked and afraid of loss.

It is a very powerful vulnerability that one must face gently and with meekness ... blessed meekness! Sooner or later the loss must be consumed if we are to live the tradition.

FINDING CAUSE December 13

Finding cause does not include analysis.

If there is something you want to trace to cause you must remain neutral and wait in neutrality...then eventually the cause will be known.

Tracing cause through analysis does not lead to the Health or the recognition of real suffering. Instead it leads to the compensations, which may appear as cause, but really do not lead to freedom and ease in the whole.

Be very careful of psychology as a spiritual tool, or a guide to find cause, as it is a man-made science with a different goal than Osteopathy. Osteopathy leads to the Spirit of Life and Health therein.

PERCEPTION December 14

Wisdom ... Discernment ... Rational Thinking

There are different kinds of "knowing" ... as a result of our educational process we are reductionistic.

Reductionism is a process that is rational and based on learned facts selected to produce a homogenized mind-set. If a patient has hypertension then it is treated in a rational manner that completely excludes the patient. The hypertension is the disease and no further diagnosis is sought. This is how medicine is practiced in most offices and it has little to do with the patient being seen as a whole within the context of an entire lifetime. People who perceive the world this way consider themselves in general to be intelligent and aware of more than the patient. Parents also use this method with their children and channel them into roles that fit the parents' ideals, leaving the child out of the picture. There is no love here.

Discernment is a different level of perception, one that listens and senses a wholeness hidden behind superficial appearances. In practice one sees past the lesion, past the personality, past the fears into a place where the true essence and Health is unveiled. This may sound like a better way to approach the patient and in a relative sense it is ... but it is still perception that has its cause or fulcrum in the observer. Discernment requires a mind that is still and alert. If the mind is not free, it will lead to an intuitive conclusion. ... It moves us closer to wholeness but can become a lesion if one begins to feel like they have insight.

Wisdom is a special form of perception of Wholeness, requiring participation, which lies beyond the polarizations possible in the above conditions. Wisdom comes from the Divine. It cannot become a skill. It never feels knowing, only loving and whole. There is no object in the mind of the seer. There is no discernment.

Wisdom is an effect of the Divine Love transmutating our senses, in the moment when we know the least. Wisdom can replace discernment if one has faith in the Divine and the patience to be neutral to all impressions previously viewed as skillful.

An understanding of these different kinds of knowing is vital to the process of finding the true self and its role in Life.

OSTEOPATHY IS — December 15

Simply put, Osteopathy is the art of using one's hands to engage a therapeutic process governed by the Health of the patient.

REST — December 16

Resisting the resistance.

What does that do?

TEMPO — December 17

The evolution of the sensorium and the faith in the Tide is a single event.

We begin the process by leading the treatment with force both manual and mental. Later, we begin to trust a little in something supernatural—as Still said in a Higher or Supreme Intelligence.

THE LESION FIELD — December 18

The idea of a lesion 'field' has been useful in understanding the dynamics of lesions as living processes. The idea that a lesion is isolated from the rest of the body does not fit very well in a general practice setting that considers the patient as a whole.

A lesion field is not restricted to tissue, nor is it restricted by fascial planes. It is spread out over a considerable area and involves all levels of function as described by Dr. Still. The lesion field is conceived by intelligent forces that are protecting the whole from losing its evolution towards perfect completeness.

The story of the lesion field begins with trauma. Dr. Fulford told us that whether the patient was in inhalation or exhalation, at the time of the trauma, would affect the patterning of the lesion. He also said that the Whole is transcendent and precognitive in its wisdom. The Wisdom sees what is coming and sets up a fulcrum that protects the Whole by organizing the stress into an isolated process—the result is the lesion field.

The geometry of the lesion field does not allow the flood-tide of the stress that insults the patient to be without limits. One can find the boundaries of the lesion field by sensing its shape rather than palpating for tissue tensions around anatomical landmarks. Once the boundaries are defined if one wishes to look at structure one may do so, although this is not necessary.

Using the boundaries of the lesion field as one's orientation, one looks for force vectors. These vectors are the matrix of the geometry of the lesion field and hold the form in an inertial dynamic that increases the lesion's stress on the whole economy of the patient as time passes. Lesions are not as static, as we first learn to think about them.

The lines of force in the vectors of the lesion field all lead to a fulcrum. During the trauma to the system, in a precise organized event of management by the wisdom indwelling in Life, these vectors emerged, channeled through the doorway of the fulcrum to form an organized field.

THE LESION FIELD — December 19

Let's review the aspects that are present in the lesion field that one can witness with listening hands:

1) Motion that is present in response to involuntary activities such as Primary and Thoracic Respiration. This motion can seem quite small but when engaged it can lead to a complete and universal treatment.

2) A sustained connection with the Whole

3) Physiological Barrier

4) Un-physiological Barrier—displacement from local midline

5) Asymmetry

6) Inertia — the persistent force that resists change, a force which grows over time, one that depletes functional reserve

7) Compression

8) A "withering field",[1] loss of a complete response to the Water of Life

1 Still page 39 Philosophy of Osteopathy

9) Loss of potency in the Fluid Drive

10) Loss of Fluid Body

11) Loss of tissue motion

12) Loss of collective neutral in tissue, fluid, and potency

13) Autonomic aberrancy—inhibition or excitation of natural state

14) Central Nervous System compromise in neurotrophic flow

15) Boundaries and force vectors

16) A direction of ease

17) A story

18) A Thread that leads to and from the Health

19) A therapeutic Stillness

20) Fulcrums of inertia and fulcrums of momentum

21) Something never seen before

THE LIMIT OF TREATMENT December 20

Still said, "your skill is proportionate to your understanding of normal." [1]

The limit in a treatment is your understanding of normal. How could this be true?

---

1 personal notes Kirksville 1967

BRAIN SAG

December 21

Brain sag is an important diagnosis to be able to feel.

It can occur from small strokes, CSF leakage which can present as severe headache, or from aging and unknown causes. We also see it sometimes during pregnancy. In the aging process the elder will feel a general weakness and memory loss. The treatment can sort out the problem and help the patient in most normal cases.

The treatment approach we present in the courses is minimal. One engages second level stillness in the cistern and waits for Thoracic Respiration to restore involuntary motion.

One can be more holistic in treatment if one finds the Health in the fluid. This is a specific place of perfect function. Then you will be drawn ... involuntarily ... into the Sea Around Us[1] and the Dynamic Stillness. This depth unites Primary and Thoracic Respirations into a single fire and can create changes that more closely merge the body and the spiritual into their original union.

The endpoint is an increase in vertical height in the fluid, an increase in fluid drive and a suspension of the cerebellum in a more natural position.

NEW HORIZONS

December 22

Our task during the journey towards Health and skill refinement is:

Be aware of things you have never seen before.

This requires a clear awareness of your personal goal and the fact that we know we have not come to the summits that Still and Sutherland traversed.

Once you recognize the event you are in and you see your interaction is a habit, then look behind the veil and see if there is another activity at a deeper level. This will reveal another landscape if... you are neutral and peacefully indifferent to the event. Do this when a treatment seems clear and is going well.

1 See Notes and Bibliography

REST December 23

In cases of severity the patient must rest for 72 hours after treatment.

This is not negotiable. One must:

Drink lots of water.

Watch dreams

And REST.

VISCERAL December 24

Visceral activity can be evaluated through involuntary motion.

Direct action is not necessary at all. Sutherland introduced a method that works very well. Find the motion in the lesion and synchronize with it, all the time being aware of the whole.

The peritoneal sac is a wonder of nature. It is worth the time it takes to read about growth and development of the sac. Notice that if the peritoneal sac is balanced then usually the viscera will follow and resume their involuntary motion secondary to Primary and Thoracic Respiration.

Retroperitoneal viscera will respond to indirect methods as well as more refined methods...BUT...make sure Thoracic Respiration is free, especially the sternal motions as described by William G. Sutherland in his teaching.
[1]

This connection, between the motion of the sternum, Thoracic Respiration, and the peritoneal sac, is vital to dynamic interchange between all the fluids of the body. How is this possible?

1 Sutherland pages 207-215 Teachings in the Science of Osteopathy

CHRIST December 25

Christmas: the birth of Christ in the stable of the heart.

The stable in the domain of poverty. The place where one finds true Shelter from the world. Poverty is empty of content.

ARCHETYPES December 26

The 'embryo' as an archetype has freed many a soul from the illusion that they have been damaged as a victim or are genetically doomed.

There is a place inside you, and behind the veil of your self-deception, that is perfect in breath, form, function and consciousness.

It is not just spirit as many would believe, but it is incarnate perfection. The embryo is the perfect incarnate being. To know this one must experience it; to experience it one must be still, quiet inside, resting, and on vacation from grief and pride.

CHRIST December 27

The days around Christmas are especially quiet.

Go outside…listen as far away as is easy…something is happening.

Christ was a real gift for mankind; his teachings, however, are difficult to follow, not as a religion but as principles. Test his words, follow them only a short way … do they work? A teacher should be tested by the student…not matching will against will, but out of respect for human limitations and what could be truth beyond our knowledge. Testing principles is the way to affirmation. It is not a challenge but an inquiry for truth.

Christ has been a part of my life and yet He is not a religion.

He is alive and waiting. He is the most feminine presence I have ever encountered.... He is not a human being as we understand them. Christ was a leader for Still and Sutherland and all my teachers. No one made a fuss about it as they genuinely were Christians ... that is, on the path to Absolute Love. Ruby was trying hard to love a man who beat her daughter. Anne was a Rosicrucian ... she lived with a genuine grief for her lost husband, you could feel it, yet she gave her children life. I never heard religion mentioned once by any of them except in personal times of strife. People like these do not grow on trees. Loving God is a good thing.

THE STAGES December 28

Student.... Apprentice.... Journeyman.... Master....

We enter the profession as students, eager to learn. There are no books per se just teachers and mentors.

Teachers have a limited forum by which to transfer experience. Courses are usually set in stone, and filled with large quantities of information.

Mentors allow us to sit beside them as they work...after a period of months or years they may trust you to be able to value what you learn and not dribble it away in conversation.

Journeymen and women are at the center of their life. They are artists and skilled practitioners who strive for more understanding.

Masters have accepted the Truth completely and function only in a moment, never doing the same thing twice ... including how they think. As teachers they are protecting the legacy with brevity and meaning. That is: yes is yes and no is no ... there are no maybes.

SILENCE — December 29

Stillness and Silence are not the same reality, even though they have the same cause.

Stillness has power. One can sense the potency of stillness as it transmutates the patient and the clinician. Silence is flowing, alive with movement. Sometimes silence has the feeling of soft rain. Sometimes it has the feeling of a river flowing in eternity…the scene is silent yet there is incarnate motion… one feels the movement of creation. This is important.

REST — December 30

Sutherland said "It is the Stillness of the Tide that we see."[1]

And in that all weariness is transmutated.

OSTEOPATHY — December 31

Think about this simple fact: normal involuntary motion is the essence of well-being.

One function that we often miss is the involuntary motion of the attention and its meaning. Let your attention REST….just let it be. It may begin to show new landscapes.

1 Sutherland Contributions of thought

Bibliography

Andrew Taylor Still

Autobiography of Andrew T. Still
With a History of the Discovery and Development of the Science of Osteopathy
Revised Edition Published by the Author, Kirksville, MO 1908
Copyright 1908 by A.T. Still
Reprinted 1981, 1989,1994,1996,2000
American Academy of Osteopathy
3500 DePauw Boulevard, Suite 1080
Indianapolis, IN 46268

The Philosophy and Mechanical Principles of Osteopathy
Hudson-Kimberly Pub. Co. Kansas City MO 1902

Philosophy of Osteopathy
A.T. Still Kirksville Mo 1899,
Reprinted by the Academy of Applied Osteopathy and the American Academy of Osteopathy

Osteopathy Research and Practice
A.T Still Kirksville Mo 1910
Originally published by the author
Reprinted by The Journal Printing Co. Kirksville Mo
Reprinted by Eastland Press Inc

William Garner Sutherland, D.O.

Teachings in the Science of Osteopathy
Edited by Anne Wales, D.O., Rudra Press
Reprinted by the Sutherland Cranial Teaching Foundation, Inc.

Osteopathy in the Cranial Field
Original Edition
Compiled by the Osteopathic Cranial Association
Edited by Harold Ives Magoun, D.O.
Approved by WG Sutherland
Second printing 1997 Sutherland Cranial Teaching foundation

Contributions of Thought, The Collected Writings of William Garner Sutherland D.O.
Pertaining to the Art and Science of Osteopathy Including the Cranial Concept in Osteopathy covering the Years 1914-1954
Edited by Adah Strand Sutherland and Anne L. Wales, D.O., Second Edition
The Sutherland Cranial Teaching Foundation 1988, Rudra Press

The Cranial Bowl, A Treatise Relating to Cranial Articular Mobility Cranial Articular Lesions and Cranial Technic
Extracts from Lectures Relative to the Cranial Concept
Published as an aid to continued study
Free Press Company

Rolin E. Becker, D.O.

Life in Motion, The Osteopathic Vision of Rolin E. Becker
Edited by Rahel E. Brooks, M.D.
Rudra Press

Rollin Becker's "1965 Sutherland Memorial Lecture" was reprinted in Life in Motion and before that in the newsletter of the Cranial Academy in December of 1965

Laurens van der Post

The Lost World of the Kalahari
Harvest Book, Harcourt Brace and Company, San Diego, New York, London.

Venture to the Interior
Random House

Rebecca Conrow Lippincott, D.O. And Howard A. Lippincott, D.O.

A Manual of Cranial Technique
Academy of Applied Osteopathy
Reprinted by The Cranial Academy

Dr. Thomas F. Schooley

Osteopathic Cranial Association Journal, 1953

Notes

Some Notes from Dr. Jealous

Dr. Jealous, over his 30 years in practice, spent hours reading, re-reading, thinking and working through ideas from Drs. Still and Sutherland and his teachers. The words and ideas that he developed over time come from the texts written by Dr. Still and Sutherland and from conversations with their students -- Dr. Jealous's teachers. In the first draft, of *An Osteopathic Odyssey,* there were multiple sections in which Dr. Jealous noted that his ideas were summaries, or paraphrasing of ideas from the texts written by Dr. Sutherland or Dr. Still. Only on rare occasion, in this text or in classes, will Dr. Jealous comment that an idea he has is new, or in fact was his own idea. The following sections contain notes or ideas from a variety of sources.

Preface

Dr. Jealous paraphrases Still, from page 19 of *Philosophy and Principles of Osteopathy* "An Osteopath answers questions by his learning. He proves what he says by what he does."

"Dig on" is widely quoted and repeated and is attributed to Sutherland who tells a story of going back to dig for more potatoes and finding little seedlings. This story is referenced in the second edition of COT on page 43, 183, 295, 301,* Page 183 is the beginning of a talk in which Sutherland tells the story and references this metaphor many times.

In the sentence "open secret of the Master Mechanic who is close at hand and breathing for the love that binds our wounds and our community" from the preface, Dr. Jealous uses some words from Still that cannot be attributed to a single place in Still's writing but the reader familiar with A.T. Still's language will recognize the use of his words.

"Not yet known" is attributed in idea to Lauren's Van Der Post but it is not a direct quote.

June 18th
A note from Dr. Jealous: When I first introduced the idea of sensing, some of Osteopathic reductionists accused me of occult activity. This happened several times with Sutherland Cranial Teaching Foundation board members. As a result of the challenge, I turned to the Oxford English Dictionary, which was clear on the difference between palpation and sensing:

Palpate: "mid 19th century: from Latin palpat- 'touched gently', from the verb palpare. Examine (a part of the body) by touch, especially for medical purposes.
Sensing: late Middle English (as a noun in the sense 'meaning'): from Latin sensus 'faculty of feeling, thought, meaning', from sentire 'feel'. The verb dates from the mid 16th century. Perceive by a sense or senses, Be aware of.

July 2nd
Dr. Jealous summarizes the following quotation from Chapter 10 in the Philosophy of Osteopathy: "The soul of man with all the streams of pure living water seems to dwell in the fascia of his body."
October 16th Note from Dr. Jealous: There is no single reference for all this material. It is from 20 or 30 sources both observational and in literature. One article you might enjoy is "The Proceedings of the Royal Society of Medicine, vol.62, dec.1969, page 1301, Section on Radiology.

Notes from the Elders

Since it's inception, Osteopathy has been passed on through the oral tradition, rather than the written word. Today, Osteopathic Universities teach both Allopathic and Osteopathic medicine, and offer a limited curriculum of traditional Osteopathic history, philosophy and practice. True students of Osteopathy, still to this day, must learn Osteopathy in the same way that their elders did; by sitting in offices of more experienced Osteopathic physicians and by watching and participating in clinical treatments over many years. The other primary means of learning this science, historically and at this time, is in small study groups, lectures, meetings and correspondence, through letters and phone calls (and now emails). There are perhaps a dozen texts written about Osteopathy by the elders of the tradition including those listed in the biography as well as a few others. However, many of the quotations in "Osteopathic Odyssey" are from notes, or letters, or were passed on orally to Dr. Jealous by his teachers and mentors. These mentors are referenced here:

Anne Wales D.O.

Dr. Wales graduated in 1926 from the Kansas City College of Osteopathy and Surgery. She met Dr. Sutherland in 1943 and began working with the Lippincott Study Group in New Jersey. Later she and her husband Chester Handy D.O. formed their own study group, the New England Cranial Study Group. Dr. Wales continued to meet with study groups in New England and practiced Osteopathy well into her 90's, during which time she was a teacher and mentor of Dr. Jealous. She is the editor of Teachings in the Science of Osteopathy, and with Adah Sutherland she also edited Contributions of Thought, The Collected Writings of William Garner Sutherland. The following sections in An Osteopathic Odyssey, contain quotes from Anne Wales, which Dr. Jealous collected while attending the study group around 1988:

April 19th
Ann Wales reporting from Dr. Sutherland.

Other sections which are referenced to Ann Wales:

July 30th
September 26th
September 27th
September 29th
October 2nd

Ruby Day, D.O.

Ruby Day was a student of Dr. Sutherland's for nearly twenty years. She also taught cranial courses with him. She was a country doctor who treated every patient. When the direct action model was promoted after Will's death she retired from the SCTF. Dr. Jealous studied with Ruby Day traveling to her home and working under her tutelage for nearly 20 years. She was dear friends with Anne Wales. After Ruby's death, Dr. Jealous formed a study group with Anne Wales and continued with Dr. Wales until her death.

The following sections contain quotes from Ruby Day that were recorded in personal notes by Dr. Jealous during these teaching hours:

January 22nd
This quote was from Dr. Sutherland through Dr. Day and told to Dr. Jealous in 1981 "there is foam on the surface of the sea, the wind will come and disperse it."

April 19th
Ruby reporting Dr. Sutherland.

July 18th
This quote was from Dr. Sutherland, through Dr. Ruby Day, to Dr. Jealous

September 27th
Last line in this section is attributed to both Anne Wales and Ruby Day

October 3rd
"You are not the last station on the railway, doctor!"
(1982)

Other sections which are referenced to Ruby day:
January 24th
August 16th
September 4th
October 30th

Rollin Becker, D.O.

Dr. Rollin E. Becker, D.O. was a student of Dr. W.G. Sutherland and himself had many students during his nearly 60 years of clinical practice. A teacher, mentor and colleague to Dr. Jealous, Rollin Becker inspired him and worked with him for many years. Their correspondence took place in letters and meetings. The quotations in this text from Dr. Becker are from the personal correspondence between these Dr. Jealous and Dr. Becker. Some of Rollin Becker's words were complied by Rachel E. Brooks MD in *Life in Motion* and *The Stillness of Life*. Dr. Jealous noted in his writing that he did not read the texts compiled by Rachel Brooks but that his quotes are from meetings and conversations that he personally had with Rolin. The following sections contain quotes from Dr. Becker:

January 2nd
"All one does is begin a treatment."

February 5th
Previously referenced quotation from 1965 Sutherland Memorial lecture

February 9th
"The fulcrum is established pre-cognitively by the Tide before the impact of the insult."

October 4th
"If you are only aware of the head, you are limited."

October 5th
"The physician's role is to save man." This section is based on a conversation with Rollin in November 1986, the quote is Rollin's.

October 6th
Conversation with Rollin Becker.

November 30th
The treatment begins when the will of the patient surrenders to the will of the Tide."

December 17th
"Boss" was a term Rollin Becker used this term to describe the relationship he had with the Tide.

Bill Johnson, D.O.

January 8th In a personal conversation, this teaching concept from Ann Wales and Ruby Day was confirmed when Bill Johnson told Dr. Jealous that the endpoint of a Functional method treatment was when the whole soma was moved by Thoracic Respiration.

Other Notes Regarding Quotations from texts by Still and Sutherland

January 2nd
"I bind the wound and God heals it" attributed to Greek physician Galen, was quoted in the forward of *Philosophy of Osteopathy* by A.T. Still. The foreword was written by the Committee of Publication of the Academy of Applied Osteopathy.

January 15th
Withering fields is quoted by Sutherland on page 188 and 213 in Contributions of Thought. In this text it is attributed to Still. Still wrote it in his Philosophy of Osteopathy on page 39.

January 22nd
" A little learning is a dangerous thing; Drink deep or taste not the Pierian spring." Attributed to Alexander Pope and reprinted on the dedication page of the first edition of *Osteopathy in the Cranial Field.*

January 20th
The first paragraph of this section is a quotation directly from Dr. Still, however the words have been changed slightly and some words have been omitted. For the exact text see Still page 16-19 *Philosophy of Osteopathy*.

January, 27th September 16th and December 21st
Dr. Sutherland discusses the experience of the sea and the tide in his lecture on August 4th 1951 printed in *C.O.T.* He references Rachel L. Carson's text *The Sea*

Around Us. It is mentioned other times in his texts as well, including on page 300 of *C.O.T.* The metaphor of the 'sea around us' is a recurrent theme and teaching in traditional Osteopathy and the Biodynamic Model.

January 30th
*Dig on - see note above in Preface
April 23rd, October 9th
The word *groundswell* appears multiple times in *Teachings in the Science of Osteopathy*, see pages 16, 17,32 and 174.

April 24th and July 16th and October 9th
"When all the fulcrums are synchronized there will be peace and harmony" Sutherland was quoted saying this and Dr. Jealous references that it was passed on to him by John Harakel. John was Rolin's son in law and President of the SCTF when Dr. Jealous joined the board.

June 1st
Be still, and know that I am God;
I will be exalted among the nations,
I will be exalted in the earth!

This quotation, from Psalm 46:10 New King James Version (NKJV)was referenced by Sutherland in the second edition of *Contributions of Thought* in the "Final Lecture, April 25th 1948" page 209

August 7, November 23rd and December 2nd. The House under the Sea is an image mentioned many times by Dr. Jealous in his lectures and manuals, as well as this text. Dr. Jealous states that Sutherland asked his wife to paint a picture of a house under the sea, transparent to the motion of Primary Respiration and explains that this was a summation of his years of research.

July 17th
This is from the Andrew Taylor Still Papers which are available online. It is in an article called "Message from the Old Doctor to Osteopathic Truth" and is reported to

be written by Still on October 15th 1916 intended for publication in a monthly journal. "The Osteopath is one who has a mechanical knowledge of the human body, when normal and when abnormal; and he should know how to adjust all variations from the normal."

August 1st
Withering fields is quoted by Sutherland on page 188 and 213 in *Contributions of Thought*. In this text it is attributed to Still, Sutherland also attributes it to Still in C.O.T. Still wrote it in his *Philosophy of Osteopathy* on page 39.

August 15th
"Every drop knows the tide" In the second edition of *Contributions of Thought*, on page 255, Dr. Sutherland quotes Rachel L. Carson's the Sea Around Us: There is no drop of water in the ocean, not even the deepest parts of the abyss, that does not know … the tide.
September 28th
The story about the scales is a paraphrasing of a story reproduced in *Contributions of Thought*, 2nd edition on page 346.

October 8th
On page 349 in the 2nd edition of *Contributions of Thought* Sutherland says "Hold the reciprocal tension membrane and the fluctuation of the fluid at the balance point. You can feel them tug-tug-tug."

October 22nd
"highest known element." Sutherland references this from A.T. Still multiple times in *C.O.T.*

October 23rd
Dr. Sutherland is referencing Still in Chapter XXVI Page 302 in the revised edition of his Autobiography says about Osteopathy, "No human hand framed its laws"

BIODYNAMICS OF OSTEOPATHY BOOK SERIES

This series of books grew organically from sets of handouts written by Dr. Jealous and given to students during the courses taught by him and his teachers. After many years he collected the handouts together and created individual course manuals, which he added to and rewrote many times. After several more years they evolved further into books. It is recommended that you read the whole series in order, as each book builds on the understanding from previous books. Prior knowledge of osteopathy is assumed, and it also recommended that you seek knowledgeable and experienced teachers and mentors to help you experience the full depth of the information given.

The full series is as follows:

Phase One is about involuntary motion, which is motion present in the whole and in the lesion. We learn to synchronize with the breathing of Primary Respiration before we approach any treatment. This synchronization is the key to working with stable rates and not irritating the system. The principle of synchronizing with a healthy aspect of the patient suffuses the whole teaching program. This synchronization shifts our awareness to a different level of receptivity, which allows us to see Primary Respiration rather than the lesion field, and this eventually leads us to an understanding of the intention of Primary Respiration.

Phase Two is about communication with the natural laws of healing that surround activity at 2 to 3 cycles per minute. We synchronize with the breathing of Primary Respiration and also add the skill of sensing the fulcrum, the Stillness through which the breathing creates form and function. It is a different kind of synchronization from that in Phase One, shifting our awareness more deeply. As this occurs, the treatment automatically expresses itself. The end point of treatment, when compared with Phase One, reveals several differences. We find this kind of synchronization works exclusively with the fluid body and the outcome of treatment is more complete than when working with tissue alone.

Phase Three is centered around the activities of the Long Tide (100 second cycle). We explore an indwelling therapeutic force already present in the lesion field. We learn that the dural system is not made-up of three sickles but rather a series of folds in a sac, arising during growth and development. We see the relationship between the upper and lower dural sacs, awakening us to the independence of two separate tentorium cerebelli. We discover that zone D, the horizon, and the Wire (along which the Long Tide moves during its intended therapeutic course) are all linked as natural laws pertaining to this level of Primary Respiration.

Phase Four focuses on the Midline, a place where the spatial relationships are expressed as a whole. It synchronizes and centers us in such a way that we become aware of Zone D and the Dynamic Stillness. The Third Level Stillness in Phase Four is different from the Stillness in the other Phases – we are centered by the Stillness at the center of creation. Our intention is replaced by the intention of the Tide which can facilitate our spiritual path.

Phase Five is about *the face*. As we approach the face, we use all of the principles that we have learned in Phase One, Two, Three, and Four. We work with automatic shifting and notice differences from how the face is viewed by older models within Osteopathy in the Cranial Field. As we synchronize with the therapeutic presence of the Long Tide we see what we can learn about the face from that landscape. We also work with Seams, Dynamic Stillness, and Ignition.

Phase Six is a continuation of our journey into the Wholeness that generates life and delivers therapeutic forces that transmute lesions once Neutral is expressed. It is a mixture of activities centered around the outside presence of Primary Respiration as something that is a non-biological force and that has a persona. We will also continue to explore seams and then move on to the extremities, first in the embryological terms and then as Sutherland taught them in his work called PowerPoints. Phase 6 is a time to build your understanding of the Tide and refine your skills.

Phase Seven highlights the Health. Dr. Still's famous comment "Find the Health; anyone can find disease," has plagued many minds over the last century. We come to the clear vision of several indwelling aspects of the Health: Love ... liquid light ... and a diamond matrix. A approach to the terminally ill and dying patient is addressed. In the somatic sensation of the Tide passing through the House Under the Sea, our awareness is transmuted by the Health. The lesion is seen as a precognitive act of the Health. Thoracic Respiration, Primary Respiration, and Ignition are as One. The landscape is vast ... and the principles of healing are even more substantial than we have previously experienced.

Phase Eight is a deeper exploration of seams, balanced rhythmic interchange, and the Flame of Intention as a therapeutic modality. Phase Eight is the culmination of our awareness of Wholeness, and ultimately brings us to the Divine Presence, Unconditional Love and Oneness. The living Tide dominates the awareness while forms move to the background. One feels the Breath of Creation in oneself as the Center of Wholeness. One feels the Unfoldment of oneself as one is Created. Our consciousness is a gift; we do not own it and if we try to control it we lose Wholeness.

Phase Nine is when we are able to fully evaluate and treat the Central Nervous System and the Eye. We also address Fire and the therapeutic modality of the Shakedown. True action is moved from Love and makes our perception exist. This Love is self-emptying and by its nature allows us to Serve as part of the Perfect. Perception can be used to Serve something other than ourselves. We have attempted to enter this balance point between the Perfect and the Disease ... it is a point where the whole of everything is suspended by Love as it works to incarnate the Complete. In the balance point of everything is The Intention of the Tide following the movement of the distortion back to a True relationship with the Blueprint of Life.

Pediatrics One explores how children grow as a whole, not in parts as we sometimes believe. Children live in the Direction of Ease of motion present in their fluid metabolic fields, otherwise they get uncomfortable and require assistance. Does your treatment directly support the whole, or does it assume to support the whole? We realize children are not adults and cannot be treated as adults are. We approach the therapeutic modality of the "Meeting Place", prenatal and postnatal periods, the treatment of the pelvis during pregnancy, fetal malposition and labor.

Pediatrics Two is where we deepen in the perceptive awareness necessary to approach the treatment of children. We deepen in our appreciation of Wholeness, the three levels of Stillness and the "Meeting Place". We approach "Desert Neutral", where therapeutics pass into the neutral substance, and a mystery unfolds as the breath of Divine love cascades as a therapeutic force across a night desert landscape, filling and leaving behind no visible effects. We further address treatment of the pelvis and the uterus during pregnancy. We explore thoracic and Primary Respiration in children, and the Family Circle.

Pediatrics Three is where we continue to study the therapeutic Flow of Attention. We deepen in Third Level Stillness and the Meeting Place. The Meeting Place is easily misinterpreted ... our observer must be so still and neutral that the process can be seen as it happens. The central nervous system in the child can be finally approached for evaluation and treatment. We explore teething and also the "locked up head". We use the therapeutic modality of the Flame of Intention, and its connection to the Breath of Life. Everything is transparent to the Breath of Life.

ABOUT THE AUTHOR

James Jealous, D.O. (1943–2021), was an osteopathic physician, teacher, and writer. His life's work was founding and developing **Biodynamics of Osteopathy**, a unique methodology he established within the field of osteopathy, following the lineage of Dr. A.T. Still and Dr. W.G. Sutherland.

He was born in Saco, Maine, and since his father was an osteopathic physician, he was around osteopathy from an early age. He studied at Kirksville College of Osteopathic Medicine in Missouri (now the A.T. Still University of Health Sciences), graduating in 1970. He then set up practice in rural Maine as an osteopathic primary care physician.

Over time, Dr. Jealous saw parallels between the work of embryologist Dr. Erich Blechschmidt and that of osteopathic physician Dr. William Garner Sutherland. This inspiration led him to create his own body of work. In the early 1990s, he began teaching "A Biodynamic View of Osteopathy in the Cranial Field," which, as he developed his specific methodology, was refined to "Biodynamics of Osteopathy."

A deeply spiritual person, he felt most at home in the natural world and was an avid fisherman and hiker.

For more information, please visit:
https://BiodynamicsOfOsteopathy.com

www.ingramcontent.com/pod-product-compliance
Lightning Source LLC
LaVergne TN
LVHW020325220926
848484LV00001BB/3
* 9 7 9 8 2 9 5 7 5 0 4 4 1 *